100 CASES
in Acute Medicine

REMOVED
FROM
STOCK

Kerry Layne
Core Medical Trainee, Guy's & St Thomas' NHS Foundation Trust, London, UK

Henry Fok
Academic Clinical Fellow, Guy's and St Thomas' NHS Foundation Trust, London, UK

Adam Nabeebaccus
Specialist Registrar, Cardiology, King's College, London, UK

100 Cases Series Editor:
Professor P John Rees MD FRCP
Professor of Medical Education, King's College London School of Medicine at Guy's, King's and St Thomas' Hospitals, London, UK

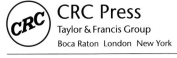

CRC Press
Taylor & Francis Group
Boca Raton London New York

CRC Press is an imprint of the
Taylor & Francis Group, an **informa** business

CRC Press
Taylor & Francis Group
6000 Broken Sound Parkway NW, Suite 300
Boca Raton, FL 33487-2742

© 2012 by Kerry Layne, Henry Fok and Adam Nabeebaccus
CRC Press is an imprint of Taylor & Francis Group, an informa business

No claim to original U.S. Government works
Printed on acid-free paper

Printed and bound in India by Replika Press Pvt. Ltd.

International Standard Book Number: 978-1-4441-3519-0   (Softcover)

**Library of Congress Cataloging-in-Publication Data and
The British Library Cataloging Data Are Available**

**Visit the Taylor & Francis Web site at
http://www.taylorandfrancis.com**

**and the CRC Press Web site at
http://www.crcpress.com**

CONTENTS

Contents

ACKNOWLEDGEMENTS

Dr Mark Kinirons, 'for making us laugh during times of stress'.

CASE 1: SHORTNESS OF BREATH AND A COUGH

History

A 64-year-old Afro-Caribbean woman has presented to the emergency department. She has been feeling generally unwell for several weeks and has become increasingly breathless over the last four days. She describes a non-productive cough but denies any fevers or night sweats. Her medical history is significant for a recent diagnosis of right-sided carcinoma of breast that was treated with a lumpectomy (removal of the tumour in the breast) and a course of chemotherapy.

Examination

The woman has reduced breath sounds on the right side of her chest, with dullness to percussion. Pulse oximetry applied to her finger shows a reading of 92 per cent on room air. A chest X-ray is performed in the emergency department (Fig. 1.1).

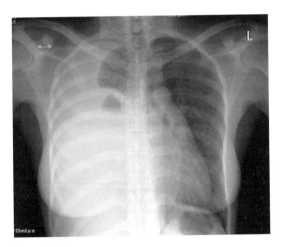

Figure 1.1

Questions

- What does the chest X-ray show?
- How would you investigate the underlying cause?
- What would be the best treatment to help this patient's symptoms?

ANSWER 1

The chest X-ray shows a large right-sided pleural effusion, as indicated by the opacification of the right lung field and loss of the costophrenic angle. This is often called a 'white-out' appearance. The mediastinum (heart, great vessels, trachea and oesophagus) has been pushed towards the left side of the chest.

A sample of the fluid is needed. Pleural fluid can be sampled using a needle (thoracocentesis or pleural tap) and then analysed. An ultrasound probe should be used to help identify exactly where the effusion is present, and then a needle can be safely inserted, ideally into the 'safe triangle' area – a triangle bordered by the mid-axillary line, the lateral border of the pectoralis major muscle, a line superior to the horizontal level of the nipple, and an apex below the axilla.

The fluid should be inspected grossly: is it blood-stained or straw-coloured? Does it appear viscous? These features will give clues to the underlying cause of the effusion.

Four types of fluid accumulate in the pleural space: blood (haemothorax), serous fluid (hydrothorax), chyle (chylothorax) and pus (empyema).

Effusions can be classed as *transudates* or *exudates*, based on their levels of protein and lactate dehydrogenase (LDH). Transudates are caused by systemic conditions that alter the balance of pleural fluid production and resorption, such as heart failure, renal failure and cirrhosis, and tend to have lower levels of protein and LDH. Exudates are caused by more local conditions, such as bacterial infection or malignancy, and tend to have higher protein and LDH levels.

In this case, the patient has a history of breast cancer, so the fluid in her pleural space is likely to be a malignant effusion, and is likely to be an exudate. It may be that her breast cancer has spread, so further tests will be needed to identify whether this is the case.

With smaller effusions, a thoracocentesis may remove enough fluid to improve symptoms; but in a case like this, where there is a large volume of fluid, a chest drain should be inserted.

Pleural effusions can recur, particularly malignant ones. Patients who develop malignant effusions despite optimal treatment of the malignancy may be referred for a pleurodesis. This involves inducing scarring of the pleura, either chemically or surgically, so that they adhere together to prevent fluid re-accumulating.

 KEY POINTS

- Patients with a pleural effusion will typically have reduced breath sounds and dullness to percussion with decreased vocal resonance and tactile fremitus on the affected side.
- Pleural fluid can be sampled via thoracocentesis, but a chest drain may be needed for large effusions.
- Patients who develop malignant effusions may be referred for a pleurodesis.

History

A 32-year-old woman suffered a collapse while exercising at a gym. Her friends described the woman falling to the floor. This was followed by twitching of her arms and legs and then a period of being unrousable. The woman remembered nothing following her arrival at the gym, and was confused and drowsy for 10 minutes following the event. She has bitten her tongue but did not lose continence. She has no past medical history of note, takes no regular or recreational drugs, and there is no family history of seizures. She has an extensive travel history, having backpacked around Asia and trekked through Nepal where she stayed in hostels and ate street food five years ago. She describes being 'completely fit and well' prior to the event.

Examination

The woman is alert and fully orientated and there are no significant findings on examination. An HIV test is negative. A CT head scan initially showed a cystic ring-enhancing lesion. Two days later, an MRI head scan was performed (Fig. 2.1).

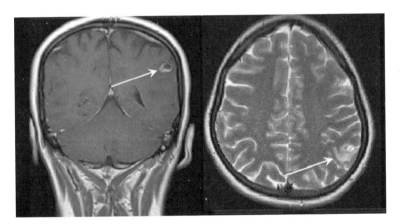

Figure 2.1

Questions

- In view of the history and scans, what is the most likely diagnosis?

ANSWER 2

This woman has presented with a generalized seizure. Having a first fit in adult life is unusual, so underlying pathology must be considered, such as a space-occupying lesion or a cerebral bleed, as well as metabolic disturbances.

The CT scan showed a lesion in the left parietal lobe with a central focus and ring-enhancement. The differential diagnosis of ring-enhancing cerebral lesions in patients with intact immune systems typically includes primary or secondary tumours and pyogenic abscesses. In immunocompromised patients, consider also *Toxoplasma* infections, lymphoma and cerebral tuberculosis. This patient's HIV test was negative and she had normal blood counts.

The MRI scan shows the lesion in better detail, revealing the classic 'dot-in-hole' appearance that is associated with neurocysticercosis. This is the most common parasitic infection of the central nervous system and the leading cause of adult-onset seizures in the developing world. The infection has a complex cycle and begins with humans ingesting raw or undercooked pork from pigs infected with *Taenia solium*. These humans can develop tapeworm infections and shed embryonated eggs in their faeces. In areas with poor hygiene facilities or where human waste is used as a fertilizer, these embryonated eggs can be ingested, leading to cysticerci developing in all tissues, particularly in the brain, eyes and subcutaneous tissue.

This patient should receive anti-helminth medication. Most patients will remain free of seizures once the underlying structural lesions are broken down. This may take some time following anti-helminth medication, and some people will need to remain on anti-epileptic drugs for months to years.

 KEY POINTS

- Neurocysticercosis is the most common cause of adult-onset seizures in the developing world and should be considered in all atypical first fits.
- Always take a full social history from a patient, including travel details, as this can provide vital information regarding exposure to environmental and infectious diseases.

CASE 3: DIARRHOEA FOLLOWING ANTIBIOTICS

History

A 68-year-old man is an inpatient on the stroke unit. He recently commenced a second course of intravenous antibiotics for aspiration pneumonia. He initially improved clinically, and the consolidation on his chest X-rays was clearing up. Then he spiked a temperature and complained of abdominal pain. His nurse reports that he has opened his bowels eight times in a short period, passing large volumes of greenish, liquid stool each time.

Examination

The patient's abdomen is generally tender throughout and bowel sounds are hyperactive. The abdomen appears distended. He is febrile (38.0°C), tachycardic (110/min) and hypotensive (88/44 mmHg). An abdominal X-ray is performed (Fig. 3.1).

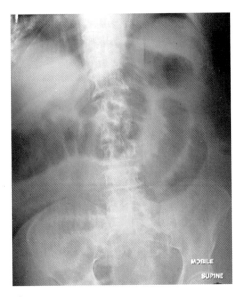

Figure 3.1

Questions

- Why has the patient developed diarrhoea?
- What does the X-ray show?
- What is the next step in management?

This man has developed profuse diarrhoea following on from a lower respiratory tract infection that is being treated with multiple antibiotics. The diarrhoea could be related to intolerance of antibiotics or a simple gastrointestinal (GI) infection, but in this case the symptoms are more worrying. The patient has signs of sepsis (fever, tachycardia, hypotension) and is passing large volumes of liquid stool, so it is important to consider pseudomembranous colitis.

Clostridium difficile is an anaerobic bacterium that can reside in the gut normally, but can also be acquired in institutions such as hospitals and residential homes. When the gut has normal intestinal flora present, *C. difficile* rarely causes problems. This patient has had multiple courses of antibiotics recently, which will have depleted the normal spectrum of bacteria living in the gut. The *C. difficile* survives and multiplies. This releases toxins that cause abdominal pain, bloating and diarrhoea. This leads to symptoms of pseudomembranous colitis.

The X-ray shows prominent, dilated loops of large bowel with evidence of mucosal oedema seen as thickened haustral folds. These features suggest that the patient may have toxic megacolon.

This patient also shows signs of septic shock. Early treatment with intravenous fluid rehydration is necessary. If the patient is not cardiovascularly stable, senior help should be sought immediately.

The microbiology department should be notified of your suspected diagnosis and stool samples must be sent to look for *Clostridium difficile* toxin. If the patient is well, fluid rehydration may suffice. Sometimes, oral antibiotics targeted at the *C. difficile* may be needed. Mild infections may be treated with oral metronidazole; more severe infections, or those that fail to respond to metronidazole, can be treated with vancomycin. Antibiotics to treat pseudomembranous colitis should be given only following the advice of a microbiologist.

If toxic megacolon is suspected, the patient may be at risk of visceral perforation. A nasogastric tube should be sited to allow GI decompression, and the patient should be made 'nil by mouth'. The surgical team on-call will need to review the case.

Drugs that slow faecal transit (e.g. loperamide) should be avoided. They are thought to prolong exposure to the *C. difficile* toxin and worsen the prognosis. There is some evidence that probiotic drinks taken concurrently with antibiotics may reduce the risk of *C. difficile* infection.

Infective spores are present in stool, so effective hand-washing and barrier nursing is necessary to prevent spread of *C. difficile* among staff and patients.

KEY POINTS

- Antibiotics deplete the natural gut flora and place patients at risk of superadded infections by bacteria such as *Clostridium difficile*.
- Suspect pseudomembranous colitis in patients who have used antibiotics and present with profuse diarrhoea and other abdominal symptoms.
- *C. difficile* is highly infective. Hand hygiene and barrier nursing should be maintained at all times.

CASE 4: SWOLLEN GLANDS AND HEARING IMPAIRMENT

History

A 19-year-old medical student has been brought to the emergency department by his flatmates who are concerned that he has become progressively unwell over a period of 5 days. He initially had symptoms of a mild coryzal illness, with a sore throat, headache and cough. For the past 72 hours he has been intermittently febrile, complaining of right-sided earache and deafness, and nausea. His sore throat is worsening and he feels as though his 'glands are up'. He describes being unable to swallow food or fluids. He has no medical history and did not experience any significant childhood illnesses, although he did not receive all his normal childhood vaccinations owing to parental concerns regarding immunizations.

Examination

This young man is febrile and tachycardic. There is marked cervical lymphadenopathy and his right ear is erythematous and swollen. He has painful bilateral testicular swelling. An audiogram shows significant hearing loss in the left ear (Fig. 4.1): the straight line represents normal hearing at particular frequencies and anything below this would be classed as abnormal.

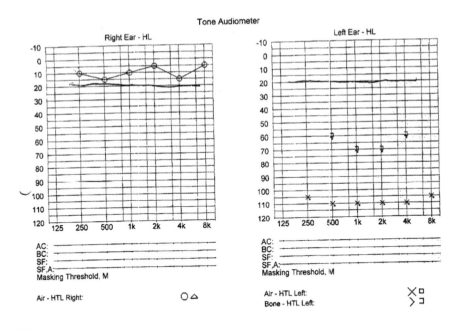

Figure 4.1

Questions

- What condition does this young man have?
- How would you treat the patient?

ANSWER 4

The patient has mumps, which is a viral illness. Patients typically develop painful swelling of the parotid glands, which initially starts as a sore throat and can progress to odynophagia (pain on swallowing). The illness is often mild and self-limiting in younger children but tends to be more serious in teenagers and adults. As well as parotitis, patients also complain of headache, fevers and orchitis. Around 30 per cent of males will develop orchitis and half of these will be left with minor testicular atrophy. Rarely, post-pubescent males can be left infertile as a result of prolonged orchitis.

Although less common, hearing loss can be one of the more serious consequences of mumps infection. Mumps is the most common cause of unilateral acquired sensorineural hearing loss in children and young adults worldwide, so physicians should advise patients to report any changes in their hearing. Occasionally, the disease can progress to encephalitis, but this is very uncommon.

The incubation period for mumps is usually 14–18 days from exposure to onset of symptoms. The infectious period is from 3 days before until approximately 9 days after onset of symptoms. The more serious complications of mumps, such as meningitis, encephalitis and orchitis, may occur in the absence of parotitis, which can delay accurate diagnosis of the clinical syndrome.

Outbreaks remain frequent, particularly among students. As recent uptake in the MMR vaccination programme has fallen over recent years, diseases like measles and mumps are becoming increasingly common.

Treatment is primarily supportive, so symptoms of pain are controlled with analgesia and fevers are treated with paracetamol. If there is evidence of hearing impairment, oral steroids should be started urgently. This patient complained of hearing loss and an audiogram was performed, which showed that he had left-sided sensorineural deafness as a result of his infection.

 KEY POINTS

- Mumps infections are becoming increasingly common, particularly now that there has been reduced uptake of the MMR (measles, mumps, rubella) vaccine.
- Suspect mumps in a patient who presents with parotitis and fever.
- Patients should be made aware that hearing loss can occur as a result of mumps infection, and to be vigilant for any symptoms. Start steroid therapy if there are any signs or symptoms of sensorineural hearing loss.

CASE 5: NOSE BLEED (EPISTAXIS) FOLLOWING AN OPERATION

History

An 85-year-old woman suffered a fall, as a result of which she fractured her left neck of femur and was admitted to the orthopaedic ward. She underwent a successful operation. Since her medical history included hypertension and chronic renal impairment, her team were aware that low-molecular-weight heparin (LMWH, e.g. enoxaparin) should be avoided; hence heparin was used postoperatively to prevent thrombus formation. Four days later the patient is complaining of a nosebleed that does not seem to be stopping.

🔍 INVESTIGATIONS

Blood count at admission:

		Normal range
White cells	9.9	$4-11 \times 10^9$/L
Haemoglobin	12.8	13–18 g/dL
Platelets	350	$150-400 \times 10^9$/L

Repeat count after the nosebleed:

		Normal range
White cells	10.2	$4-11 \times 10^9$/L
Haemoglobin	11.8	13–18 g/dL
Platelets	90	$150-400 \times 10^9$/L

Questions
- Why might the patient's platelet count be falling?
- Should you stop the heparin?

ANSWER 5

This woman needs to be investigated for heparin-induced thrombocytopenia (HIT). This is a condition that typically develops 4–10 days after commencing treatment with heparin, and is more common with unfractionated heparin than with LMWH. IgG antibodies to heparin develop that activate platelets and cause clot formation. This causes the platelet count to fall and also predisposes patients to thrombosis.

A HIT screen can be performed, sending blood samples for an ELISA test to identify heparin-binding antibodies. Doppler ultrasound scans of the legs tend to be performed routinely in anyone suspected of having HIT, as deep vein thromboses are very common in this condition. The graph (Fig. 5.1) shows the patient's platelet count during her hospital stay.

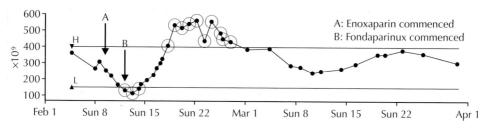

Figure 5.1 Graph to show platelet levels during admission

Patients with HIT have a low circulating platelet count, which can predispose them to bleeding, but they paradoxically have an increased risk of thrombosis due to platelet activation. Anticoagulation is needed to prevent clot formation. Warfarin is contraindicated, as patients with HIT are predisposed to warfarin-related necrosis. Patients are usually switched to a factor Xa inhibitor, often an alternative LMWH or similar compound, that is less commonly associated with HIT. An example is fondaparinux.

Some studies have shown that up to 15 per cent of patients treated for more than 5 days with unfractionated heparin or LMWH will develop a 50 per cent reduction in their baseline platelet count. The majority of these cases will not be due to HIT, but the condition is always something that you should consider.

 KEY POINTS

- HIT is the development of thrombocytopenia following treatment with heparin and typically presents 4–10 days after the first dose.
- It predisposes to thrombosis, so treatment requires anticoagulation with an agent that will not further reduce the platelet count.
- Some patients treated for more than 5 days with unfractionated heparin or LMWH will develop a reduction in their baseline platelet count. The majority will not be due to HIT.

History

An 89-year-old woman was admitted to hospital with new-onset confusion. Her daughter had noticed that she had become increasingly forgetful over the past week and now was no longer orientated to time and place. Her medical history was significant for hypertension, for which she took bendroflumethiazide. She was normally independent in her activities.

Examination

The patient's urine dip was found to be normal and her inflammatory markers were not elevated.

INVESTIGATIONS		
		Normal range
Sodium	114	135–145 mmol/L
Potassium	3.8	3.5–5.0 mmol/L
Urea	6.8	3.0–7.0 mmol/L
Creatinine	98	60–110 µmol/L

The patient was given 4 L of 0.9% saline over the next 24 hours. The following morning she became more confused, drowsy and dysarthric. When a neurological examination was performed, she had reduced power throughout all muscle groups and there was increased tone and brisk reflexes in the lower limbs. Her blood tests showed a sodium level of 138 mmol/L.

Questions

- What was the probable cause of the woman's initial confusion?
- Why has the patient deteriorated?

ANSWER 6

The patient was hyponatraemic at presentation. A sodium level of less than 125 mmol/L is considered a severe hyponatraemia.

Hyponatraemia is the most common electrolyte abnormality and is more frequent in elderly patients. Symptoms tend to be very non-specific and can include nausea, vomiting and confusion. If sodium levels drop low enough, neurological features, such as muscle cramps and seizures, can develop. Serum sodium levels and osmolality are usually tightly controlled by homeostatic mechanisms. As hyponatraemia progresses, patients can develop marked neurological symptoms as sodium leaves the bloodstream and the change in osmotic pressures leads to the development of cerebral oedema.

This woman takes a thiazide diuretic, which acts on the distal convoluted tubule, inhibiting the sodium–chloride symporter so that sodium resorption is reduced. This is a common cause of sodium loss in patients.

Patients with any form of fluid overload, such as in congestive cardiac failure or nephrotic syndrome, can develop a hypervolaemic hyponatraemia.

Hypovolaemic hyponatraemia can occur when patients are losing fluid though vomiting and diarrhoea, not drinking sufficient volumes of water, or becoming volume deplete, for example due to the use of diuretics. Hypovolaemia stimulates antidiuretic hormone (ADH) release and subsequent water retention, which leads to a dilutional hyponatraemia.

The syndrome of inappropriate ADH release (SIADH) occurs when there is excessive release of ADH, causing water retention and, as stated above, a dilutional hyponatraemia. This can be due to damage to the posterior pituitary gland, infections such as meningitis or brain abscesses, and small-cell lung cancers that secrete ectopic hormones.

The likely diagnosis here is that the woman has developed central pontine myelinolysis. This is a condition that can occur when serum sodium levels are rapidly altered, as the osmolar pressures shift, destroying the sensitive myelin sheath around the neurons. Demyelination can lead to severe neurological damage and the sudden alteration in osmolar pressures can cause cerebral haemorrhage. When treating hypo- and hypernatraemia, you should aim to correct sodium levels by no more than 10 mmol/L per day.

 KEY POINTS

- Hyponatraemia is a common electrolyte abnormality that can cause symptoms of confusion and non-specific malaise.
- Patients using diuretics should be monitored for hyponatraemia.
- Rapid correction of hyponatraemia can lead to central pontine myelinolysis, a life-threatening neurological condition.

History

A 19-year-old student has been admitted to hospital after being found unconscious in her room in university halls of residence. Her room-mate told the paramedics that she had recently failed her end-of-year exams and had ended a long-term relationship earlier that week. She is not known to have any medical history and took occasional painkillers for a knee injury. She was found with several empty packets of paracetamol around her. A suicide note was discovered next to her.

Examination

The student is drowsy but responsive. She admits to taking thirty 500 mg paracetamol tablets and eight 30 mg codeine phosphate tablets with a bottle of wine approximately 4 hours earlier. Observations: temperature 36.4°C, heart rate 80/min, blood pressure 110/70 mmHg, respiratory rate 12/min, SaO_2 96 per cent on room air.

INVESTIGATIONS		Normal range
White cells	7.0	$4–11 \times 10^9$/L
Haemoglobin	14.0	13–18 g/dL
Platelets	290	$150–400 \times 10^9$/L
Sodium	139	135–145 mmol/L
Potassium	4.9	3.5–5.0 mmol/L
Urea	5.5	3.0–7.0 mmol/L
Creatinine	75	60–110 μmol/L
C-reactive protein	<5	<5 mg/L
Bilirubin	20	5–25 μmol/L
Alanine aminotransferase	35	8–55 U/L
Alkaline phosphatase	80	42–98 U/L
Albumin	45	35–50 g/L
INR	1.1	0.9–1.1

Questions

- What are the consequences of a paracetamol overdose?
- How should this young person be managed acutely?

ANSWER 7

Paracetamol overdose is the leading cause of acute liver failure in the United Kingdom. Paracetamol is metabolized to N-acetyl-p-benzoquinoneimine (NAPQI), which depletes the liver's glutathione stores. Glutathione is an antioxidant and protects the hepatic cells from damage. High levels of NAPQI can build up after a paracetamol overdose and subsequently lead to liver failure. Liver failure can develop over hours, or even days. In this case, the patient has also taken opioid medication (codeine phosphate), which may further impair hepatic function.

In some centres, activated charcoal may be given if the patient presents within an hour of taking the overdose. This is a very porous substance and can adsorb substances such as paracetamol, reducing the levels that enter the bloodstream.

Over the first 24 hours, patients can experience nausea and sweating. Blood tests should be sent to monitor the liver function, and they classically show a hepatitic picture with raised transaminases. Liver synthetic function should be monitored closely. The liver produces coagulation factors, and measuring the international normalized ratio (INR) will indicate how effective the liver is at synthesizing these products. A persistently high INR is an indication for a liver transplant. Renal function should also be closely monitored, as an acute kidney injury can occur.

After 3–5 days, patients are at risk of hepatic necrosis. Patients can present with sepsis, impaired clotting function and multi-organ failure.

Patients should have regular observations performed and be kept in a bed where they can be monitored. Intravenous fluid rehydration should be given. In addition to the aforementioned blood tests, blood glucose checks should also be performed, as patients can become hypoglycaemic in liver failure. Serum paracetamol levels should be taken to confirm the diagnosis and help guide treatment.

The mainstay of treatment is N-acetylcysteine, which replenishes the stores of glutathione and prevents further liver damage. This treatment can be very effective if given within 8 hours of the overdose. Some people can have an anaphylactoid reaction to N-acetylcysteine, so the person must be very closely monitored.

In the longer term, the patient should have a psychiatric review to assess her risk of further suicide attempts and to identify an underlying depressive illness.

 KEY POINTS

- Paracetamol overdose is the leading cause of liver failure in the UK.
- Patients should be treated with fluids and may require N-acetylcysteine therapy depending on their serum paracetamol levels and the timing of the overdose.
- Ultimately, multi-system failure can develop, particularly if the patient presents to hospital more than 8 hours after the overdose took place. A liver transplant may be necessary.

CASE 8: LYMPHADENOPATHY AND MALAISE

History
A 19-year-old woman has presented to the emergency department complaining of fevers and malaise after returning from a holiday in South Africa two weeks earlier. Over the preceding 3–4 days she noticed a rash and sore throat and is now feeling generally tired and unwell. She has no significant medical history and does not take any regular medications or recreational drugs. She does not smoke, nor drink alcohol. She admits to several episodes of unprotected sexual intercourse with a man she met in South Africa.

Examination
The young woman is febrile and tachycardic. Her heart sounds are normal, her chest clear and her abdomen soft and non-tender. She has widespread lymphadenopathy: the lymph nodes are 2 cm in diameter and are soft and tender on palpation. There is an erythematous, maculopapular rash covering her trunk. Observations: temperature 37.8°C, heart rate 98/min, blood pressure 110/88 mmHg, respiratory rate 16/min, SaO_2 99 per cent on room air.

INVESTIGATIONS		
		Normal range
White cells	14.0	$4–11 \times 10^9$/L
Haemoglobin	15.0	13–18 g/dL
Platelets	100	$150–400 \times 10^9$/L
Sodium	133	135–145 mmol/L
Potassium	3.7	3.5–5.0 mmol/L
Urea	4.5	3.0–7.0 mmol/L
Creatinine	77	60–110 µmol/L
C-reactive protein	78	<5 mg/L

Questions
- What are the possible diagnoses that you should consider?
- If the patient's HIV test comes back as positive, what should you do next?

ANSWER 8

This woman is likely to have a viral illness, considering her history of fevers, rash and sore throat.

Infectious mononucleosis (glandular fever) secondary to Epstein–Barr virus is a common illness in young adults, presenting with fever, rash and lymphadenopathy following on from a sore throat. A monospot antibody test can rapidly identify a patient with current Epstein–Barr infection. Blood tests show a lymphocytosis, and often an acute hepatitis, from which patients will gradually recover over the following weeks.

Human immunodeficiency virus is another infection that must be considered in those with fevers, night sweats and significant lymphadenopathy, particularly if the patient has risk factors, such as intravenous drug use or unprotected sexual intercourse. The patient should be counselled for an HIV test, explaining to her both the potential benefits and disadvantages of receiving a positive diagnosis. She should be advised that it can take up to 3 months for the HIV test to become positive and that, if her test is negative now, she should still be retested 3 months later.

The differential diagnosis should also include infections (e.g. tuberculosis), as well as haematological malignancies (e.g. Hodgkin's lymphoma). Detailed history-taking will allow you to identify the most likely diagnoses and test for these as necessary.

In addition to the full blood count, tests should be done to measure the CD4 and CD8 counts and the HIV viral load, as well as the renal and hepatic functions. A routine chest X-ray should be performed to look for signs of infection or cavitating lesions suggesting tuberculosis infection (more common in HIV-positive patients).

T-lymphocytes express either CD4 molecules, which initiate an immune response to bacteria, viruses and fungi, or CD8 molecules. The HIV virus binds to CD4 molecules and rapidly reproduces. As people seroconvert in the weeks following infection, they develop symptoms consistent with a viral illness, such as fever and lymphadenopathy. The CD4 cells are gradually destroyed by the virus and, after several years, patients begin to develop infections.

The patient should be referred to the local HIV team who can take a focused history and identify any specific treatment she will need. She should undergo testing for other sexually transmitted infections, such as syphilis, gonorrhoea and Chlamydia. Contact tracing should also be encouraged, so that anyone else at risk of contracting HIV from the patient, or the person who passed the infection to the patient, can be identified. They will assess the patient and consider antiretroviral treatment.

 KEY POINTS

- Consider HIV infection in patients presenting with symptoms such as fever, rash, lymphadenopathy or arthropathy.
- Patients with a positive HIV test should be referred to an HIV team who can monitor CD4 counts and consider introducing antiretroviral therapy.

CASE 9: THE ILL RETURNING TRAVELLER

History

A 46-year-old man has presented to the emergency department complaining of fevers, vomiting and general malaise. He describes experiencing fevers and rigors every 8–12 hours for the past three days. He feels weak and tired and has vomited several times. He has recently returned from a holiday in Ghana where he took part in a camping trip. He was previously fit and well with no medical problems and no regular medications.

Examination

This man is febrile (39.7°C) and tachycardic (100/min). He looks pale and his mucous membranes are dry. His abdomen is soft but tender at the left upper quadrant, where splenomegaly of approximately 8 cm is palpable. He has multiple skin lesions around his ankles, which he attributes to mosquito bites.

Questions

• Considering the possible diagnosis, what investigations should you request?
• How should this man be treated?

ANSWER 9

The patient describes swinging pyrexias and has moderate splenomegaly. He has recently returned from Ghana and has many mosquito bites on his extremities. It would be useful to ask the patient whether he was taking antimalarial prophylaxis. The clinical features fit a diagnosis of malaria and appropriate tests should be requested to look for this.

A full blood count may show anaemia (predominantly due to red blood cells being destroyed by malaria parasites) and a thrombocytopenia. Renal and liver functions may also be deranged. A blood film will confirm the presence of malaria parasites, identify the species of parasite and measure parasite levels.

The treatment will depend on which type of malaria the patient has. *Plasmodium falciparum*, with a high parasite count, will need treatment with intravenous quinine followed by oral doses. Five per cent dextrose may need to be given, as blood glucose levels can fall in these patients. Other types of malaria, such as *Plasmodium malariae*, *P. vivax* and *P. ovale*, are more benign and can usually be managed with a short course of oral antimalarials.

 KEY POINTS

- Malaria should be suspected in patients with an appropriate travel history who present with fevers and rigors.
- In patients with suspected malaria, blood should be sent for thick and thin blood films, looking for the presence of the parasites.
- Once a parasite has been identified, treatment advice can be sought from an infectious diseases specialist to guide further management.

History
An 88-year-old woman has been admitted to hospital after her daughter visited and found her to be confused. For the past three days the patient has complained of feeling tired and has become increasingly disorientated. She was normally relatively fit and well, lived alone and was independent for all activities of daily living (ADLs). On direct questioning, she describes symptoms of urinary frequency and dysuria.

Examination
This woman is febrile (39.4°C) and tachycardic (108/min). She is a slim woman, weighing approximately 55 kg. She has mild suprapubic tenderness. Her abbreviated mental test (AMT) score is 6/10.

INVESTIGATIONS		
		Normal range
White cells	18.0	4–11 × 10⁹/L
Neutrophils	16	2–7 × 10⁹/L
Haemoglobin	13.0	13–18 g/dL
Platelets	305	150–400 × 10⁹/L
Sodium	138	135–145 mmol/L
Potassium	3.9	3.5–5.0 mmol/L
Urea	12	3.0–7.0 mmol/L
Creatinine	140	60–110 μmol/L
C-reactive protein	94	<5 mg/L
Urine dip: 3+ leucocytes, nitrites positive		

Questions
- What is the likely underlying cause of this patient's confusion?
- Over the first few hours she remains tachycardic (100/min) and her blood pressure is now starting to fall. What should be done?
- Her heart rate remains high despite initial treatment and her blood pressure continues to fall (70/30 mmHg). Her urine output is initially good (60 mL/h) but begins to tail off (20 mL/h). How will you manage her now?

ANSWER 10

The patient is febrile and tachycardic, features that can suggest an infection. She has additional symptoms that suggest that the infection could be in her urinary tract: dysuria and urinary frequency along with suprapubic tenderness. Her urine dipstick shows nitrites in the urine. Bacteria present in the urine can produce enzymes that convert urinary nitrates to nitrites that show up on the dipstick test. Elderly people, particularly females, are more prone to urinary tract infections and often present with confusion.

The patient is showing signs of sepsis, probably a urosepsis. She should be treated according to the Surviving Sepsis guidelines (http://www.survivingsepsis.org) with broad-spectrum intravenous antibiotics as soon as possible. Her tachycardia and hypotension suggest that she will need to be given intravenous fluids. A catheter will probably need to be inserted in this case to monitor her fluid balance status, although generally this should be avoided wherever possible as catheters can introduce a further source of infection.

Blood cultures should be taken – preferably before antibiotics are given, but without delaying their administration. Her urine should also be sent to the laboratory for microscopy, culture and sentitivities. She can be started on a broad-spectrum antibiotic, but if a specific bacterium is grown and the antibiotic sensitivities become available, her antibiotic can be changed to a more targeted therapy.

The patient is haemodynamically unstable. She should be given a fluid challenge, by administering a bolus of a colloid fluid, such as 250 mL of gelofusine. She should be monitored for signs of response to this, such as an increase in blood pressure, normalization of her heart rate or an improvement in urine output. She may need to be assessed for a bed on a high-dependency unit where inotropic drugs can be given along with close monitoring of her fluid status via a central venous line to improve her heart rate and blood pressure.

The patient's daughter should be informed that her mother is very unwell and may not survive. If the patient is well enough, her wishes regarding intubation and resuscitation should be discussed with her.

 KEY POINTS

- Urinary tract infections can often present with non-specific symptoms, such as confusion and general malaise, particularly in elderly patients.
- Early treatment according to the Surviving Sepsis protocol is key to ensuring patients have the best chance of surviving a serious infection.

History

A 28-year-old pregnant woman who is at 34 weeks' gestation presents to the emergency department complaining of a headache. She feels nauseous and has noticed some ankle swelling over recent days. This is her first pregnancy and she has been well up until this point.

Examination

This woman's heart rate is 70/min but her blood pressure is 160/90 mmHg on three different readings, taken 10 minutes apart. Her heart sounds are normal and her chest sounds clear. A full neurological examination is significant for 6 beats of clonus at both ankles. The symphysis–fundal height is 34 cm (normal for the gestation) and the presentation is cephalic. The fetal heart rate is 130/min. Her urine has been dipped and shows the presence of protein.

Questions

- What condition could this pregnant woman be suffering from?
- How would you manage the patient?

In a pregnant woman, an elevated blood pressure (>140/90 mmHg) or a rise in baseline systolic blood pressure of >20 mmHg and/or diastolic blood pressure of >10 mmHg, along with the presence of 300 mg protein in a 24-hour urine collection, should alert you to the possibility of pre-eclampsia. Sustained clonus (>5 beats) is one of the neurological signs that develop in pre-eclampsia.

Pre-eclampsia is a potentially life-threatening condition that affects women who are at more than 20 weeks' gestation.

If pre-eclampsia is not managed, the condition can progress to eclampsia, with a high risk of seizures, cerebral haemorrhage and adult respiratory distress syndrome.

Early support from the obstetrics team will be key in managing this patient. Her blood pressure will need to be controlled to prevent seizures and intracerebral haemorrhage. Labetalol is a commonly used antihypertensive in these situations. An infusion of labetalol can be set up and titrated according to the patient's blood pressure. Magnesium sulphate is often given to help prevent seizures.

Steroids should be given to promote fetal lung maturity in case early delivery is needed. If the condition continues to progress, delivery of the fetus will be necessary. Signs of pre-eclampsia typically settle within 48 hours of delivery.

 KEY POINTS

- Pre-eclampsia should be suspected in a pregnant woman in the second or third trimester who presents with hypertension and evidence of proteinuria on urine dipstick.
- This life-threatening condition should be managed in a hospital setting with involvement from obstetricians.
- A labetalol infusion may be required to manage hypertension, and magnesium may need to be given to prevent seizures.
- Ultimately, if pre-eclampsia progresses, early delivery of the fetus may be necessary.

CASE 12: EPIGASTRIC PAIN AND VOMITING

History

A 55-year-old man has presented to the emergency department with abdominal pain and vomiting. He says the pain came on gradually yesterday. The pain is dull and constant, in the epigastrium and the centre of the abdomen and radiating to his back. He has had multiple previous admissions to hospital, which were primarily related to alcohol excess. He admits to drinking around 50 units of alcohol per week and has been drinking particularly heavily over the last fortnight. He smokes 20 cigarettes per day. Apart from some admissions related to trauma there is no significant medical history. His mother had type 2 diabetes but there is no other family history. He is divorced, lives alone in a flat and is unemployed.

Examination

This man's upper abdomen is very tender but soft. His bowel sounds are normal. His heart rate is 110/min, blood pressure 112/74 mmHg.

INVESTIGATIONS		
		Normal range
White cells	19.4	4–11 × 10⁹/L
Haemoglobin	13.1	13–18 g/dL
Platelets	160	150–400 × 10⁹/L
Sodium	142	135–145 mmol/L
Potassium	3.9	3.5–5.0 mmol/L
Urea	8.4	3.0–7.0 mmol/L
Creatinine	85	60–110 μmol/L
C-reactive protein	140	<5 mg/L
Amylase	1200	30–110 U/L
Glucose	14.7	3.5–5.5 mmol/L

Questions

- What is the most likely cause of this man's abdominal pain and vomiting?
- How would you confirm your diagnosis, and what treatment could you give?

The man has features of pancreatitis, which classically presents with upper abdominal pain radiating though to the back, and vomiting. The serum amylase level is often raised and the patient may have signs of an inflammatory response, such as a fever and an elevated white cell count. The patient may be jaundiced.

There are numerous factors that predispose a person to developing pancreatitis, but gallstones and alcohol misuse are the leading causes in the UK.

Acute pancreatitis can be life-threatening, with mortality rates of up to 10 per cent.

The clinical features plus the elevated serum amylase level should be enough to diagnose acute pancreatitis. An abdominal ultrasound scan will show inflammation and oedema of the pancreas as well as the presence of gallstones and can exclude other forms of abdominal pathology if the diagnosis is in doubt. A CT scan will also show inflammation of the pancreas.

The patient will need analgesia for his stomach pain; usually regular intravenous paracetamol is commenced. He should be kept 'nil by mouth' and intravenous fluids should be given. Although there is little supporting evidence for efficacy, intravenous antibiotics are often given. A nasogastric tube may be sited to decompress the stomach and reduce the activity of the pancreas.

As patients can go on to develop an acute kidney injury or even acute respiratory distress syndrome, blood tests should be performed at least daily to monitor the full blood count, renal function, liver function and coagulation. An arterial blood gas should be performed to check that the patient is not hypoxic and to monitor the lactate level, which can become elevated in sepsis or severe inflammation. As the pancreatitis progresses, patients can develop hyperglycaemia due to impaired insulin production by the pancreas. In this case the patient's high blood glucose level may be related to his pancreatitis or possibly undiagnosed type 2 diabetes mellitus (note the family history). Hypocalcaemia may also become a problem, as the inflamed pancreas generates increased levels of free fatty acids that chelate calcium salts, which then precipitate in the abdominal cavity.

In severe cases, surgical intervention may be needed to remove necrotic pancreatic tissue or to remove gallstones.

KEY POINTS

- Pancreatitis usually presents with upper abdominal pain radiating through to the back, and vomiting.
- Risk factors include gallstones and alcohol misuse.
- Acute pancreatitis can be life-threatening. Patients should be kept 'nil by mouth' with intravenous fluids and analgesia. Very close monitoring of heart rate, blood pressure, fluid status and oxygenation will need to be carried out. Surgery may need to be performed.

History

A 22-year-old man has been admitted to hospital with severe pain in his legs. He is known to have sickle cell disease and says that his pain is typical of his sickle crises. He was initially given opiate analgesia and intravenous fluids, and after 24 hours his pain has largely settled. He now complains of shortness of breath.

Examination

This young man is visibly dyspnoeic and has coarse crackles at both lung bases. His SaO_2 is now 87 per cent on room air.

INVESTIGATIONS		
		Normal range
pH	7.43	7.35–7.45
PO_2	7.4	9.3–13.3 kPa
PcO_2	3.1	4.7–6.0 kPa
Lactate	2.7	<2 mmol/L
HCO_3	24	22–26 mmol/L
Base excess	+1	−3 to +3 mmol/L
Saturation	87%	>94%

Questions
• How would you interpret the blood gas results?
• What is the probable diagnosis?

ANSWER 13

The arterial blood gas results demonstrate type 1 respiratory failure. The patient is hypoxic and is hyperventilating to try to improve his oxygenation. He is therefore blowing off more carbon dioxide, which is why the PCO_2 level is low. He is probably having a sickle cell chest crisis.

When a patient is experiencing a sickle cell crisis, the misshapen sickle cells occlude the small blood vessels and cause hypoxia and tissue damage. When the sickle cells infiltrate the lungs, this can result in a sickle cell chest crisis.

He will need urgent treatment with antibiotics and intravenous fluids. He should be given oxygen to increase his saturations to above 94 per cent. An urgent chest X-ray should be performed. He will need close observation and may need to be transferred to a high-dependency unit.

If the crisis is not improving and the blood continues to sickle, the patient should be given a blood transfusion to introduce normal red cells to the circulation. Alternatively, if the haemoglobin level is too high to allow a transfusion to be carried out safely, an exchange-transfusion may be carried out, whereby the patient's own blood is removed while new blood is transfused.

This condition can be life-threatening, so early involvement of senior medical doctors and possibly the high-dependency or intensive care teams may be necessary.

 KEY POINTS

- A sickle cell chest crisis should be suspected in patients with known sickle cell disease who develop hypoxia.
- A chest crisis can be fatal, so a patient should be reviewed early for antibiotics, intravenous fluids, oxygen and possibly a blood transfusion to try to improve the hypoxic tissue damage.

CASE 14: CHEST PAIN RADIATING TO THE BACK

History

A 74-year-old woman has presented to the emergency department with central chest pain radiating through to her back. This has lasted for 4 hours. She describes the pain as tearing in nature and scores it as 10/10 in severity. Her medical history is significant for hypertension, for which she takes regular bendroflumethiazide tablets. She takes no other medication.

Examination

This elderly woman is clearly uncomfortable, despite opiate analgesia being given. There is a loud, early diastolic murmur which is loudest at the aortic region. There is a collapsing pulse. Observations: heart rate 120/min, blood pressure 102/50 mmHg in her left arm and 80/38 mmHg in her right arm. A chest X-ray is shown in Fig. 14.1.

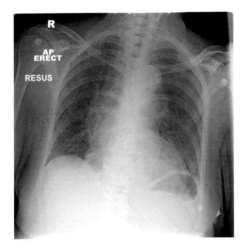

Figure 14.1

Questions

- What does the chest X-ray show?
- What is the likely diagnosis?
- How would you treat this woman?

ANSWER 14

Tearing chest pain radiating to the back should make you suspicious of an aortic dissection. This occurs when the inner lining of the aorta shears away from the vessel wall and blood flows between the layers, separating them. This can lead to aortic rupture, which has an 80 per cent mortality rate.

When the ascending thoracic aorta and/or the aortic arch are involved, this is referred to as a type A dissection, whereas type B dissections involve the descending thoracic aorta. The disparity in blood pressure between the arms indicates that the arch is involved.

There is a widened mediastinum on the chest X-ray. This can suggest that there is dissection of the thoracic aorta. The clinical signs of differing blood pressure in each arm, tachycardia and aortic regurgitation (early diastolic murmur in aortic region, collapsing pulse) are compatible with this diagnosis.

There is little you can do medically for this patient. You should ensure that she has good intravenous access and that she has cross-matched blood available for transfusion. Her blood pressure and heart rate will need to be closely managed. To prevent further shearing of the aorta, her systolic blood pressure will need to be kept below 100 mmHg. An infusion of a beta-blocker drug (e.g. labetalol) is typically used to do this.

The patient will probably need a central venous line, and transfer either directly to theatre for an aortic repair or to an intensive-care unit for initial stabilization. The intensive-care team, anaesthetists and surgeons should be notified about the patient immediately. Ultimately, the patient will need an aortic repair to be done as soon as possible.

 KEY POINTS

- Central chest pain radiating to the back should alert to the possibility of aortic dissection.
- Early involvement of surgical, anaesthetic and intensive-care teams will be needed to manage the patient, who is likely to need aggressive stabilization and surgery.

History
An 80-year-old man has presented to the emergency department complaining of severe shortness of breath. He has been feeling increasingly dyspnoeic over the last fortnight and is now unable to walk even short distances before becoming short of breath, and his legs feel heavy to lift. He is short of breath at night, too, and has gone from sleeping with three pillows to sleeping upright in his chair. He has a cough productive of frothy pinkish sputum but has not experienced any fevers. He has a history of hypertension and heart problems but has stopped taking his diuretic medication recently owing to urinary frequency and occasional incontinence.

Examination
The patient is unable to speak in full sentences owing to his dyspnoea. On auscultation there are fine inspiratory crackles in the lower and mid zones bilaterally. His heart rate is 96/min, blood pressure 150/90 mmHg. A third heart sound is audible at the left sternal edge but there are no murmurs. His jugular venous pressure (JVP) is raised at 8 cm. His ankles are swollen and there is pitting oedema up to his knees. Arterial blood gas measurements show hypoxia, and a chest X-ray (Fig. 15.1) shows bilateral fluffy areas consistent with pulmonary infiltrates.

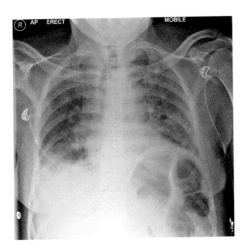

Figure 15.1

Questions
- Why has the patient become short of breath?
- What would be the appropriate management?

ANSWER 15

The patient has developed pulmonary oedema. He is known to have heart failure but this has worsened over the past 2 weeks. He has stopped taking his diuretic because of the increased urinary output that resulted from the medication. This has led to fluid overload, as evidenced by his right-sided signs of elevated JVP and peripheral oedema and the fine crackles in the lungs suggestive of pulmonary oedema.

He should be given oxygen via a facemask to improve his hypoxia and feelings of dyspnoea. A catheter should be inserted to monitor his urine output accurately and allow regular assessment of his fluid balance status.

A loop diuretic (e.g. furosemide) will need to be given to offload the fluid in the lungs. This can be either a one-off (stat) dose or a continuous infusion titrated in line with the patient's blood pressure. Furosemide will cause the kidneys to excrete large volumes of fluid via the urine. The reduction in circulating fluid volume may lead to a reduction in blood pressure, so this should be monitored carefully. Diuretics should be given intravenously initially. This is because the bowel can become oedematous in states of fluid overload, and gastrointestinal absorption is therefore reduced.

Glyceryl trinitrate (GTN) can be given as an infusion in place of furosemide and will act in a similar way to offload excess fluid through vasodilatation.

If the patient remains uncomfortably dyspnoeic, a small dose of opiate analgesia (e.g. morphine) can be given to reduce the respiratory drive.

For patients whose blood pressure is low, meaning they cannot tolerate a furosemide or GTN infusion, or those who remain hypoxic despite the above medical treatment, non-invasive ventilation (NIV) can be beneficial. NIV can redistribute fluid in the lungs and open up collapsed alveoli through positive pressure. This reduces the work of breathing and can improve the cardiovascular status by reducing the venous return and afterload.

Patients with heart failure that has not responded to diuretics should be assessed for NIV in a ward-based or a high-dependency unit setting.

 KEY POINTS

- Clinical signs of congestive cardiac failure include fine late inspiratory crackles in the lung bases, added heart sounds, an elevated JVP and peripheral oedema.
- Acute treatment usually consists of oxygen, intravenous furosemide and catheterization to monitor fluid balance. A small dose of morphine may be given to improve symptoms of dyspnoea.
- For patients who do not improve with diuretics, non-invasive ventilation may be needed to redistribute fluid in the lungs.

History
An 18-year-old woman on holiday from Greece is brought to hospital by her friends, suffering from severe abdominal pain. The pain came on gradually throughout the day and she is now in too much pain to walk unaided. She has been vomiting for the past few hours. She says she has experienced episodes similar to this over the last 2–3 years but they have usually settled down eventually. On direct questioning, she states that her cousin also suffers from similar intermittent episodes of abdominal pain.

Examination
This young woman is febrile (38.1°C) and looks pale. Her abdomen is diffusely tender and she shows signs of guarding and rebound tenderness. She has an appendicectomy scar in the right iliac fossa. The examination is otherwise unremarkable.

Questions
- What is the likely underlying diagnosis affecting this young woman and her cousin?
- How would you manage her, in both the short and the long term?

ANSWER 16

This woman gives a classic history of familial Mediterranean fever (FMF). Patients present with fevers and usually with abdominal pain that mimics peritonitis on examination. Joint pains, pleuritis and pericarditis are also common during flares of FMF.

Familial Mediterranean fever is a condition that is inherited in an autosomal recessive pattern. A mutation in the *MEFV* gene is responsible.

The acute management of FMF is usually supportive. Intravenous fluids and simple analgesia are usually enough to help the patient feel better until the attack passes. Unfortunately, doctors often diagnose appendicitis during the first attack and patients can go on to have unnecessary appendicectomies.

Colchicine, a drug usually given in gout and other rheumatological conditions, is often given prophylactically to reduce the frequency of attacks. The underlying mechanism of colchicine in reducing attacks is not known. The drug is often poorly tolerated.

Patients with FMF can go on to develop amyloidosis, a condition where abnormal proteins build up in the kidneys, heart and lungs leading to disease.

The diagnosis can usually be made with a history of recurrent attacks, particularly if other family members have already received a diagnosis of FMF. If the diagnosis is in doubt, genetic studies can be carried out to identify the mutated *MEFV* gene.

KEY POINTS

- Familial Mediterranean fever is an autosomal recessive disorder that typically affects people with a Mediterranean ethnic background.
- Sufferers present with recurrent episodes of inflammation, usually abdominal pain, but myositis, pericarditis and pleuritis can also occur.
- Patients with FMF are often given colchicine prophylactically to prevent flares of the condition. This drug also slows the progression to developing amyloidosis.

History

A 54-year-old man has attended the emergency department with shortness of breath and a cough. He has been feeling increasingly unwell over the past 3–4 weeks. He describes fevers and night sweats, a loss of appetite and some loss of weight. He has a cough productive of grey sputum, which sometimes contains small clots of blood. He has never smoked and does not drink alcohol. There is no relevant medical or family history. He has been working for a charity in sub-Saharan Africa and returned home a few weeks ago.

Examination

This man appears cachectic. He has a low-grade fever (37.4°C). His chest has a few scattered crackles throughout the upper zones. A chest X-ray (Fig. 17.1) shows a large cavitating lesion in the right upper zone as well as some left apical zone opacification, possibly representing further lesions.

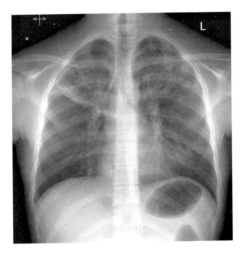

Figure 17.1

INVESTIGATIONS		
		Normal range
White cells	13.4	4–11 × 10⁹/L
Haemoglobin	14.8	2–7 × 10⁹/L
Platelets	260	150–400 × 10⁹/L
Sodium	134	135–145 mmol/L
Potassium	3.7	3.5–5.0 mmol/L
Creatinine	87	60–110 µmol/L
C-reactive protein	38	<5 mg/L

Questions

- What is the cause of this patient's cough and haemoptysis?
- What would you need to do immediately?

ANSWER 17

The patient is very likely to have pulmonary tuberculosis (TB). He has a history of fevers, night sweats and haemoptysis and the chest X-ray shows a cavitating lesion which would be consistent with tuberculosis. The patient has been living in sub-Saharan Africa, most of which has a high incidence of tuberculosis particularly related to HIV infection. He may well have come into close contact with people infected with TB.

Despite the probable diagnosis of tuberculosis, it is important to exclude a cavitating lung malignancy, which can present in a similar manner with fevers, night sweats and haemoptysis. His sputum should be sent for microscopy, culture and sensitivities and the microbiologist should be asked specifically to look for acid-fast bacilli, which signify an infection with TB. Culture of the sputum has a higher positive rate but takes 4–6 weeks.

If the sputum smear is negative for acid-fast bacilli then some further investigations will be required. He will need a CT scan of his chest and ideally a further sample will be obtained directly from the lesion, probably via fibre-optic bronchoscopy.

If tuberculosis is confirmed, the patient should be started on a multi-drug regime that will vary depending on the protocol for the region. He will be assessed by TB nurse specialists who will counsel him prior to treatment.

The presence of acid-fast bacilli in his sputum shows that the patient is a high risk for infecting others. He should initially be isolated when he begins his treatment.

The first-line drugs include isoniazid, rifampicin, ethambutol and pyrizinamide. There are various side-effects that can follow these drugs. Hepatitis can result from isoniazid, rifampicin and pyrizinamide, so liver function tests should be monitored. Isoniazid can cause a peripheral neuropathy, and pyridoxine (vitamin B$_6$) should therefore be given prophylactically to prevent this. Ethambutol is associated with ocular toxicity, so the patient must be warned to report any ocular symptoms immediately.

It is important to try to identify who the patient could have caught tuberculosis from and who he could have passed it on to. Contact tracing should be done wherever possible, ideally in the setting of a TB clinic.

Tuberculosis is more common in people who are immunosuppressed and is often present in patients who are HIV-positive. This patient should be counselled for an HIV test.

 KEY POINTS

- Tuberculosis should be suspected in anyone presenting with shortness of breath, fever, haemoptysis and weight loss.
- An important differential diagnosis to consider is lung malignancy.
- Tuberculosis should be managed by a multi-disciplinary team, including support from TB nurse specialists, respiratory physicians and community doctors.
- It is important to perform thorough contact tracing.

CASE 18: BLOODY DIARRHOEA

History
A 25-year-old man has presented to the emergency department with abdominal pain, vomiting and bloody diarrhoea. He attended a party the previous day and several other attendees had been taken ill with suspected food poisoning. He is too unwell to give any further history.

Examination
This young man appears pale and shocked. His mucous membranes are dry and he appears to be clinically dehydrated. His heart rate is 110/min, his blood pressure 90/50 mmHg.

INVESTIGATIONS		
		Normal range
White cells	18.0	$4–11 \times 10^9$/L
Haemoglobin	8.0	13–18 g/dL
Platelets	48	$150–400 \times 10^9$/L
Sodium	149	135–145 mmol/L
Potassium	7.2	3.5–5.0 mmol/L
Urea	24.5	3.0–7.0 mmol/L
Creatinine	280	60–110 μmol/L
Blood film	Fragments of red cells, suggestive of haemolysis	

Questions
- What abnormalities can be seen in the blood results?
- In view of the clinical picture and the blood results, what is the probable diagnosis?
- What would be the appropriate management?

ANSWER 18

There is a high white blood cell count, suggesting infection. The haemoglobin is low and the blood film report states that there is evidence of haemolysis (abnormal breakdown of red cells). The platelet count is also low (thrombocytopenia).

The renal tests show that the patient has an acute kidney injury. His urea and creatinine are both elevated, meaning that the patient is dehydrated and has poor renal function. The elevated potassium is particularly concerning, as this puts him at risk of developing cardiac arrhythmias.

The history of bloody diarrhoea preceding renal failure and blood tests showing a haemolytic anaemia and thrombocytopenia support a diagnosis of haemolytic uraemic syndrome (HUS). Most cases are caused by infection with the *Escherichia coli* 0157 strain of bacteria. Patients usually develop symptoms of food poisoning with bloody diarrhoea. The infection can be life-threatening: it has a mortality rate of up to 10 per cent. A further 10 per cent will develop end-stage renal failure requiring renal replacement therapy.

A patient with these features should immediately be referred to a high-dependency unit. He has an acute kidney injury and is dangerously hyperkalaemic.

The first step is to manage his hyperkalaemia. He should be given calcium gluconate to stabilize his myocardium. Insulin should be given along with dextrose to drive the potassium back into the cells. Salbutamol nebulizers can also be given to promote potassium entry into cells. Ultimately, the patient will need haemodialysis until his renal function improves.

Antibiotics are generally avoided in haemolytic uraemic syndrome as they can stimulate the release of further endotoxins.

Daily plasmaphoresis (plasma exchange to remove immune complexes) will need to be performed until the platelet count is normalizing.

 KEY POINTS

- Haemolytic uraemic syndrome is a triad of haemolysis, thrombocytopenia and renal failure, secondary to *E. coli* 0157 infection.
- Patients with HUS will probably need care in a high-dependency setting.
- Haemodialysis may be required along with plasmaphoresis.
- The pathophysiology of HUS is similar to thrombotic thrombocytopenic purpura (TTP). Please refer to Case 30 (p. 59).

History

A 56-year-old woman has been admitted to hospital after becoming drowsy and confused at work. Her daughter says that the woman has experienced several episodes of drowsiness and headaches which seemed to improve after meals. She has been rapidly gaining weight recently and has experienced intermittent palpitations. She has no medical history of note and is normally fit and well.

Examination

This woman feels cool to the touch. She is tachycardic with a heart rate of 100/min. There are no other positive clinical findings. A finger-prick blood glucose test returns 1.2 mmol/L (normal range 3.5–7 mmol/L).

Questions

- What is the probable reason for this woman's recurrent episodes of drowsiness and malaise?
- Are there any other conditions associated with this diagnosis?

ANSWER 19

The patient has recently been gaining weight. The episodes of drowsiness and headaches improve after she has something to eat. These symptoms point towards an insulinoma. This is a neuroendocrine tumour that develops in the pancreatic islets of Langerhans and produces excessive quantities of insulin. The insulin drives glucose into the cells, thus lowering the blood glucose level. Patients develop symptoms of hypoglycaemia and eventually present to hospital.

To make the diagnosis you will need to send a laboratory serum glucose sample (as finger-prick tests can be unreliable) which should come back as <3 mmol/L. Further specialist tests can then be conducted, such as insulin suppression tests to measure levels of glucose, insulin and C-peptide after a prolonged fast.

CT imaging can identify the specific location of the tumour as well as the presence of any metastases.

Medical management can involve somatostatin analogues that reduce the release of insulin, as well as careful blood glucose monitoring and the use of hyperglycaemic agents as necessary. Surgery to remove the insulinoma, wherever possible, is the treatment of choice along with targeted chemotherapy.

Approximately 5 per cent of insulinomas are associated with multiple endocrine neoplasia type 1 (MEN-1) syndrome. These patients are at increased risk of developing tumours in endocrine glands including the parathyroids, pituitary and pancreas.

 KEY POINTS

- Patients with recurrent episodes of symptomatic hypoglycaemia should be investigated for an insulinoma.
- Five per cent of patients with insulinomas have MEN-1 syndome and therefore have increased risk of developing further endocrine tumours in the pituitary and parathyroid glands.

CASE 20: PROGRESSIVE LOWER LIMB WEAKNESS

History
A 23-year-old man, who is an accountant, has presented complaining of numbness and weakness in his legs. He first noticed the symptoms two days ago, with tingling in his feet and weakness in the ankle joints. He now thinks that his legs are weak up to the thighs and has fallen over several times. He describes his legs as heavy and numb to touch. He denies any shortness of breath and feels otherwise well, although he has recently recovered from a bout of food poisoning (there are no problems with his bowels or micturition now). He has no medical history.

Examination
This young man initially had reduced sensation to both light touch and pin-prick from S1 up to the level of L2. He had reduced power throughout the lower limbs, which was worse distally. The knee and ankle reflexes were absent bilaterally. The upper limbs and cranial nerves showed no abnormalities. Twenty-four hours later he reports that his hands now feel numb.

Questions
- This patient presents with an ascending paralysis following an episode of food poisoning. What is the likely diagnosis?
- What will be your greatest concern in this patient? How will you monitor him?
- Can you think of any specific treatments for the illness?

ANSWER 20

The patient has Guillain–Barré syndrome (GBS). This is an ascending paralysis secondary to an inflammatory demyelination of the peripheral nerves. The demyelination develops in response to an immune response to a foreign antigen. There is usually no demyelination present in the central nervous tissue (brain and spinal cord).

In this case the patient has probably had an infection with *Campylobacter jejuni*, as evidenced by his episode of food poisoning. An autoimmune response is triggered, leading to GBS.

A disconcerting feature of GBS is that it can ascend to involve the respiratory muscles. This can lead to paralysis of the diaphragm muscles and subsequent respiratory arrest. Patients should be monitored closely for signs of respiratory distress and bedside spirometry should be performed every 4 hours to record the vital capacity. Clinicians should have a low threshold for intubating patients with GBS as diaphragmatic paralysis can occur rapidly over a few hours, with catastrophic consequences.

Guillain–Barré syndrome is an autoimmune condition and the mainstay of treatment is to remove the circulating autoimmune complexes. Plasmaphoresis (plasma exchange) can be performed, in addition to the administration of intravenous immunoglobulins. Supportive management with fluids and oxygen may be necessary.

Physiotherapy is key to regaining function, and involvement from occupational therapists may aid progress. Most patients return to baseline function within 1–2 months.

 KEY POINTS

- Guillain–Barré syndrome presents with an ascending paralysis that can spread to involve the diaphragm and cause respiratory arrest.
- Treatment may include plasmaphoresis and immunoglobulin administration as well as general supportive measures.
- Support from physiotherapists and occupational therapists will promote an early recovery to baseline function.

History

A 48-year-old man collapsed in the street and had what eyewitnesses confirmed to be a tonic–clonic seizure. He was admitted to hospital for further monitoring. He has never had a seizure before and has been otherwise well recently. He admitted to drinking a 75 cL bottle of vodka (30 units) daily but has been trying to cut down recently and has not had any alcohol for the past 48 hours. He initially seemed alert and orientated on arrival at hospital, but on the ward the nurses noted that he was agitated. A CT head scan was normal. The following morning he appears unwell and has vomited several times.

Examination

This man is diaphoretic and appears very agitated. His heart sounds are normal and his chest is clear. His abdomen is soft and non-tender and bowel sounds are active. He is hallucinating, describing insects covering the walls, and his hands are notably tremulous. Observations: temperature 37.0°C, heart rate 104/min, blood pressure 128/66 mmHg, respiratory rate 28/min, SaO_2 100 per cent on room air.

INVESTIGATIONS		
		Normal range
White cells	6.0	$4–11 \times 10^9$/L
Haemoglobin	14.8	13–18 g/dL
Platelets	196	$150–400 \times 10^9$/L
Sodium	138	135–145 mmol/L
Potassium	4.5	3.5–5.0 mmol/L
Urea	6.7	3.0–7.0 mmol/L
Creatinine	97	60–110 µmol/L
C-reactive protein	<5	<5 mg/L

Questions

- What are the most likely reasons why this patient had a seizure?
- What worrying features does the patient display the next morning?
- Could the deterioration have been prevented?

ANSWER 21

There can be many reasons underlying the development of seizures, but in this case we have a scenario where a man in his forties is known to misuse alcohol. He drinks around 200 units of alcohol per week (in the region of ten times the recommended maximum intake).

The first thing to rule out is an intracerebral bleed and a subsequent seizure related to this. Alcohol misuse increases the risk of intracerebral bleeds, because head injury is more likely to be sustained or as a result of deranged liver function. Sustained alcohol misuse can lead to deranged liver function and therefore reduced production of vitamin K, which is essential for normal blood clotting properties. Additionally, a long history of excessive alcohol intake can lead to cerebral atrophy, so the fragile blood vessels between the meningeal layers have to traverse a longer distance and are therefore more prone to bleeding in the event of a head injury.

The normal CT head scan in this case excludes a large intracerebral bleed. A subdural haematoma can take hours or days to develop, so this should always be considered in patients with a head injury.

Then consider that the patient could be withdrawing from alcohol. Seizures are a common way for patients with alcohol withdrawal to present. This patient reports that he has suddenly stopped drinking and has not consumed any alcohol for 48 hours. The timing of his presentation and the fluctuation in his consciousness make a seizure secondary to alcohol withdrawal likely.

The man is displaying signs of autonomic dysfunction, with tachycardia, hypertension and diaphoresis. This could all be related to the sudden withdrawal of alcohol. If not managed appropriately, the patient may develop delirium tremens, which can be life-threatening. Patients with alcohol misuse are prone to other neuropsychiatric conditions, such as Wernicke's encephalopathy, and Korsakoff's psychosis, due to a longstanding lack of thiamine (vitamin B_1).

The man should have been diagnosed as being at high risk of an alcohol withdrawal syndrome and so treated according to a withdrawal protocol. Most hospital trusts in the United Kingdom use the Clinical Institute Withdrawal Assessment for Alcohol (CIWA score) to closely monitor for signs of withdrawal. This is both an objective and subjective score, looking for signs of agitation, tachycardia and sweating, which can be early signs of withdrawal. Patients are usually given small doses of benzodiazepine as per the CIWA score. They may require regular doses of benzodiazepines, which can then be gradually reduced. People prone to alcohol withdrawal should be started on high doses of thiamine, which is usually given intravenously initially. This can help to prevent development of Wernicke's encephalopathy and Korsakoff's psychosis.

When he has recovered, the patient should be referred to alcohol support services if he wishes to continue to abstain from alcohol intake in the future.

KEY POINTS

- People withdrawing from alcohol are at high risk of seizures.
- Patients with a history of alcohol excess, who are at risk of alcohol withdrawal, should be monitored closely using a scoring system such as the CIWA score. They may require small doses of benzodiazepines to control their symptoms.

History

A 24-year-old man has been admitted to hospital with agitation and confusion. His flatmate called an ambulance because he was concerned that the man was withdrawing from γ-hydroxybutyric acid (GHB), an illicit drug that he took regularly. The man used the drug hourly in the daytime and every 3 hours at night but had not used any in the past 24 hours. He was usually fit and well.

Examination

The young man's heart sounds are normal and his chest is clear. His abdomen is soft and non-tender. A full neurological examination cannot be carried out as the man is too agitated to comply, but he is markedly tremulous. Observations: temperature 38.2°C, heart rate 114/min, blood pressure 138/84 mmHg, respiratory rate 20/min, SaO_2 99 per cent on room air.

INVESTIGATIONS		
		Normal range
White cells	10.0	$4–11 \times 10^9$/L
Haemoglobin	17.0	13–18 g/dL
Platelets	300	$150–400 \times 10^9$/L
Sodium	139	135–145 mmol/L
Potassium	4.8	3.5–5.0 mmol/L
Urea	6.8	3.0–7.0 mmol/L
Creatinine	100	60–110 µmol/L
C-reactive protein	8	<5 mg/L
Urine toxicology screen	Nil detected	NB many drugs/toxins are not screened for with this test

Questions

- How would you manage this patient's initial withdrawal?
- What other management should be considered?

ANSWER 22

Gamma-hydroxybutyric acid and its prodrug, γ-butyrolactone (GBL), are now among the most commonly used recreational drugs in UK clubs. They are central nervous system depressants and can have both euphoric and sedative effects. They are highly addictive when used in high quantities. GHB/GBL users who use large quantities of the drug may require very frequent doses and rapidly start to withdraw within a few hours without GHB/GBL.

Withdrawal from GHB/GBL can be life-threatening. It is often managed in a level 2 setting and can last for around 10–14 days. As with alcohol withdrawal, patients often require benzodiazepines, but sometimes in very high doses, so they must be monitored closely for respiratory depression. Buscopan, an antispasmodic, is also very effective in managing GHB/GBL withdrawal symptoms. As people using high volumes of GHB/GBL can rapidly deteriorate, advice from the local toxicology team should be sought wherever possible and the high-dependency team should be made aware of the patient.

Long-term support should be offered wherever possible to help patients remain free of drugs and alcohol. There are numerous addiction support groups available in the community and information about these should be given before the patient is discharged. Many hospitals have substance misuse teams that can support patients both in hospital and back in the community and provide information about accessing rehabilitation facilities.

 KEY POINTS

- GHB and GBL are now among the leading recreational drugs used in the UK.
- Withdrawal from GHB/GBL can be life-threatening and begins after only a few hours of stopping the drug in people who use large quantities.
- Advice should be sought from the hospital high-dependency team and, if available, a toxicology team.

CASE 23: UNILATERAL LEG SWELLING

History

A 38-year-old man presented to the emergency department complaining of right leg swelling and pain. The leg swelling and pain had come on progressively over the preceding 48 hours. He had no significant medical history and no previous hospital admissions. He did not take any regular medications. He had a background of intravenous drug use and injected heroin into his leg veins on a daily basis. He occasionally inhaled cocaine. He denied any history of smoking or alcohol intake. He has been admitted for observation and treatment.

Examination

On admission this man was febrile (38.4°C) and felt warm to the touch. His heart sounds were normal, with no audible murmurs and his chest was clear on auscultation. His abdomen was soft and non-tender. There were puncture wounds visible over his legs and feet, which he had used as injection sites. The lower part of his right calf was erythematous and warm to touch, with localized oedema. He was febrile and tachycardic.

Initial treatment

Intravenous antibiotics were given. Although the patient seemed to improve initially, he later developed severe pain around the site of swelling and increased erythema, which seemed out of proportion to the appearance of the leg swelling. He has become progressively more unwell over 24 hours, with fevers, tachycardia and hypotension.

Questions

- What differential diagnoses should you consider for this man?
- What would be the appropriate management?
- What is the likely cause of the deterioration with severe leg pain?

ANSWER 23

This patient has swelling and erythema of his leg, which is also warm to touch. These signs point towards an infection, such as cellulitis. Intravenous drug use can make cellulitis more likely, as injection sites become infected and nutritional intake is often poor.

A deep vein thrombosis should also be considered. Repeated venous puncture and low-grade infection promote endothelial dysfunction and higher levels of clotting factors, all leading to increased risk of embolus formation.

The examination findings should often suggest whether an infection or a deep vein thrombosis is present. In this case, the patient is more likely to have cellulitis. Blood tests will probably show raised inflammatory markers. A swab of the infected tissue should be taken, as well as blood cultures if the patient is febrile, to attempt to identify a specific bacterium causing the infection. In the meantime, a course of broad-spectrum antibiotics should be commenced. If signs of sepsis are present (fever, tachycardia, hypotension) then intravenous fluids may need to be given and the high-dependency team may need to be notified about the patient in case of deterioration. Most clinicians would also arrange a Doppler ultrasound scan of the affected limb to exclude a deep vein thrombus.

Severe pain, out of proportion to an area of infection, should always alert you to the possibility of necrotizing fasciitis. This is an infection caused by multiple bacteria, including group A *Streptococcus* and *Staphylococcus aureas* that spreads through the subcutaneous and deep tissues, releasing toxins that can lead to overwhelming sepsis. Patients often require admission to a high-dependency unit and wounds may need debriding by general surgeons or the plastic surgery team.

 KEY POINTS

- Unilateral leg swelling in a patient with intravenous drug use should prompt consideration of cellulitis or a deep vein thrombosis as possible diagnoses.
- Necrotizing fasciitis should be suspected in a patient with pain that is more severe than you would expect from the wound; but as pain is very subjective, the diagnosis can be hard to make.
- Early involvement of the surgical teams will allow debridement of the wound (if necessary) and improve morbidity.

CASE 24: VOMITING CAUSED BY NOROVIRUS

History

A 92-year-old woman was admitted to hospital with diarrhoea and vomiting. She had been vomiting for the preceding 48 hours and was now unable to tolerate any oral intake. She lived with her daughter's family, who were concerned that she was becoming dehydrated. Other members of the family had experienced similar symptoms over the last week. Her medical history includes hypertension and diet-controlled type 2 diabetes mellitus. Her drug history includes ramipril 2.5 mg once daily and bendroflumethiazide 2.5 mg once daily. She does not drink alcohol and has never smoked.

Examination

On admission, this elderly woman had dry mucous membranes and her jugular venous pulse was not visible. Her heart sounds were normal, her chest was clear and her abdomen was soft with mild, generalized tenderness. Observations: temperature 37.3°C, heart rate 98/min, blood pressure 84/40 mmHg, respiratory rate 24/min, SaO_2 98 per cent on room air. Vomit samples tested positive for norovirus.

Initial treatment

She was admitted for two days and seemed to make a good improvement. On the third day she developed shortness of breath and a cough productive of green sputum. On auscultation, she had crackles at the left base.

Questions

- How would you treat this woman?
- Why may she have developed a chest infection?

ANSWER 24

Norovirus, otherwise known as the winter vomiting bug, is an RNA virus that is a common cause of gastroenteritis. Common symptoms include vomiting, diarrhoea and abdominal pains. The virus is spread via the faecal–oral route, but can be airborne and so spreads rapidly among contacts. The virus is often self-limiting and symptoms usually resolve over several days.

Oral rehydration solutions can be useful in treatment. Patients, usually the very young and the elderly, may become severely dehydrated. The woman in this clinical scenario has features of dehydration, with dry mucous membranes and a jugular venous pulse that is hard to visualize. She also has a tachycardia and is hypotensive, again suggesting that the patient is volume depleted. Hypotension and tachycardia are features of moderate-to-severe dehydration. She needed to be admitted for intravenous fluids and monitoring of her blood pressure and heart rate as a guide to her fluid status.

She may have a chest infection, secondary to an organism acquired either in the community or in the hospital. A community-acquired lower respiratory tract infection is diagnosed when symptoms begin in the community or within 48 hours of hospital admission. When symptoms develop after 48 hours in hospital, it is more likely that a patient has acquired an infection from the unit, and this is termed a hospital-acquired pneumonia. It is important to differentiate between the two, as hospital acquired infections are more likely to be resistant to antibiotics.

In patients who are vomiting and develop signs of a chest infection, an aspiration pneumonia should be considered. This occurs when small amounts of a foreign material, such as food, liquid or vomit, enter the airway. This can cause a very serious, life-threatening pneumonia and intravenous antibiotics should be started immediately. A chest X-ray may show signs of early inflammation in the lungs, secondary to aspirated material. If there is concern about the patient's ability to swallow safely, he or she should not be allowed to eat or drink until a formal swallowing assessment has been carried out. Intravenous fluids can be used for hydration in this case.

 KEY POINTS

- Norovirus and other forms of gastroenteritis often present with vomiting and diarrhoea.
- Very young and elderly patients who are prone to dehydration may require intravenous fluids.
- Aspiration pneumonia can occur when foreign materials, such as vomit, enter the airway. This can cause a severe infection and antibiotics should be given as soon as possible.

History

An 18-year-old man presented to his GP complaining of a three-day history of fever, sore throat and a yellow discolouration of his eyes and face. He had no significant medical history and took no regular medications. There was no significant family history. He was not sexually active, did not smoke and did not drink any alcohol nor use recreational drugs. His friends and family were well and he had not travelled abroad for more than a year.

Examination

This young man was febrile but appeared comfortable at rest. His cardiovascular examination and respiratory system were normal. There was a palpable mass in the right upper quadrant of his abdomen and he had jaundiced sclera and skin. He had marked cervical lymphadenopathy. His throat was erythematous but there was no visible exudate.

Initial treatment

He was prescribed an antibiotic (amoxicillin). The following day he developed a florid rash. The rash is widespread, pink and maculopapular in nature.

Questions

- What diagnoses would you consider in this young man?
- What investigations and further treatment would you consider in this case?

ANSWER 25

This patient has a fever, sore throat and lymphadenopathy. His abdominal examination revealed possible splenomegaly also. The most likely cause would be a viral illness; and, in a young adult, infectious mononucleosis (glandular fever) caused by Epstein–Barr virus (EBV). If there is doubt, other infections, such as HIV, should be excluded.

If antibiotics (such as amoxicillin and ampicillin) are given in an oropharyngeal group A streptococcal infection, a florid maculopapular rash can develop. This is not an allergic reaction, but the antibiotics should be stopped and the patient observed.

This patient is jaundiced, so liver function tests should be requested, in addition to a full blood count, renal profile and C-reactive protein (CRP: a marker of infection/inflammation). An acute hepatitis is common in infectious mononucleosis. A heterophil antibody, such as the monospot test or Paul Bunnel test, can be up to 90 per cent specific and sensitive in diagnosing infectious mononucleosis. Antistreptococcal antibody titres (ASOT) can also be sent to look for evidence of a streptococcal infection. If the diagnosis is in doubt, consider an abdominal ultrasound scan to look at the spleen (left upper quadrant mass) and the liver (jaundice), as well as a liver screen, including hepatitis serology.

Usually, patients with infectious mononucleosis do not require hospital admission, as the disease is self-limiting; but where there is marked jaundice and deranged liver function, suggesting an acute hepatitis, a patient may need to be admitted for monitoring. Patients with hepatomegaly ± splenomegaly should be advised against participating in any contact sports for 4–6 weeks.

 KEY POINTS

- Infectious mononucleosis is a common viral disease, typically affecting young adults.
- The viral disease is usually self-limiting but patients can develop a hepatitis, which will need monitoring.
- If infectious mononucleosis is suspected, amoxicillin and ampicillin should *not* be given, as these can induce a maculopapular rash.

CASE 26: BLURRED VISION

History
A 53-year-old man has presented to the emergency department complaining of blurring of his vision and seeing 'flashing lights' in both eyes. He denies any headaches or rashes. He has experienced intermittent fevers for several days and is feeling generally unwell. He was diagnosed with HIV infection five years ago and started highly active antiretroviral treatment (HAART) six weeks earlier owing to a low CD4 count. His HIV viral load has fallen rapidly over recent weeks.

Examination
A systems examination reveals cervical lymphadenopathy. On fundoscopy, areas of infarction (white patches) and haemorrhage (red patches) are seen bilaterally. Blood tests show a high lymphocyte count.

Questions
- What could be the underlying cause for this man's visual symptoms?
- Why might he have developed these symptoms now?
- What treatment would you commence?

ANSWER 26

This patient has fevers and visual symptoms on a background of immunosuppression (HIV infection). There are many ocular infections that can affect immunosuppressed patients, including cytomegalovirus (CMV) retinitis and varicella zoster retinitis. More common ocular conditions, such as glaucoma and vitreous detachment, should be considered too. The fundoscopy findings of haemorrhage and infarction (often described as a 'pizza' appearance) are typical for CMV retinitis.

The majority of people in the UK have been infected at some point with CMV and are usually asymptomatic from this. Immunocompromised patients are at risk of developing severe CMV infections, with pathologies such as pneumonitis, gastritis, colitis and retinitis developing. CMV retinitis is an inflammation of the retina that often starts with symptoms of visual blurring and can rapidly progress to permanent visual loss if not treated urgently.

This man is at risk of CMV retinitis because he is immunocompromised from the HIV infection. His CD4 count has been low recently, which would put him at increased risk of opportunistic infections. He has recently commenced HAART, and around 4–12 weeks after commencing HAART some patients develop immune reconstitution inflammatory syndrome (IRIS), in which a rapid drop in the patient's viral load causes the immune system to recover and mount a strong response to a previously acquired infection. Patients develop symptoms of fever and inflammation, often related to underlying infections. The IRIS response can be severe and patients will often require multi-system support.

This man will need to take an antiviral agent, such as valganciclovir, which is very effective in the treatment of CMV retinitis. If treatment is not started promptly, he could lose his vision. Ideally, he should have input from a specialist HIV team and an ophthalmologist. Regular ophthalmology assessments should be carried out, even after this episode has subsided, as asymptomatic infections can recur. HAART should be continued, as this will enable the immune system to recover and reduce the risk of further opportunistic infections.

 KEY POINTS

- Immunocompromised patients are at risk of developing severe CMV infections, particularly CMV retinitis.
- Prompt treatment with antiviral agents, such as valganciclovir, could save a patient's vision.
- Patients with HIV who commence antiretroviral therapy are at risk of developing IRIS, where their immune system begins to recover and mounts a strong response against previously acquired infections.

CASE 27: RECURRING DIZZINESS WITH EXERCISE

History

An 84-year-old woman has been brought to hospital after collapsing in the street. She describes walking quickly and feeling very dizzy, then waking up a few moments later on the pavement. She has experienced several similar episodes of dizziness over recent weeks. Her medical history includes hypertension and exertional angina. She is generally fit and well, and manages to walk a mile every day with her dogs.

Examination

This elderly woman has a slow-rising, low-volume carotid pulse. On palpation, a sustained left ventricular heave is present. There is a harsh ejection systolic murmur, which is most audible at the second intercostal space in the right upper sternal border, and radiates to the carotids. The murmur is loudest in expiration. The second heart sound is soft. There is bilateral pitting oedema to the ankles. Her blood pressure is 140/100 mmHg. An ECG shows sinus rhythm with left ventricular hypertrophy (Fig. 27.1).

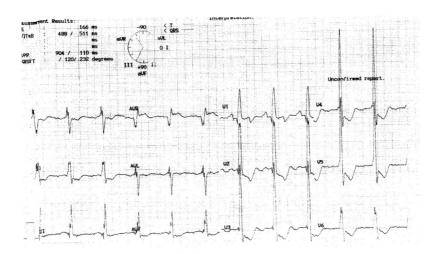

Figure 27.1 Supplied by Dr Stam Kapetanakis

Questions

- Why might this patient have collapsed?
- What management would be appropriate?

When dealing with a patient who has transiently lost consciousness (syncope), there are several possible causes to consider. The differential diagnosis should be broad as only careful history-taking and examination will allow you to establish the underlying reason for the collapse. An eyewitness account can be very helpful.

Epileptic seizures should be considered. The patient gives no history of jerking (which can also feature in syncope), tongue biting or incontinence.

The next consideration is orthostatic (postural) hypotension, whereby blood pressure drops on sitting or standing (usually by more than 20 mmHg in systolic pressure or 10 mmHg in diastolic pressure). This is more common in people who are dehydrated or suffering from heat exhaustion, or who have experienced prolonged bed rest or take medications such as vasodilators and diuretics. This woman has a history of hypertension and angina which raises this possibility.

Cardiac causes, such as an arrhythmia, should next be considered. Arrhythmias include tachycardias, such as supraventricular or ventricular arrhythmias, and bradycardias, such as sinus bradycardia or heart block. This patient did not describe any chest pain or palpitations preceding her collapse, but did feel dizzy and lightheaded, which can be features of cardiac syncope. She has an ejection systolic murmur, consistent with aortic stenosis, which can cause collapse due to limited cardiac output or arrhythmias. When exercising, the peripheral vascular system dilates to allow an increased blood flow to reach the muscles and the cardiac output usually increases. In the case of severe aortic stenosis, patients cannot increase their cardiac output sufficiently, cerebral perfusion falls and the patient collapses. This seems to be a likely cause for this patient's collapse.

In all patients who have collapsed, an ECG should be performed to identify arrhythmias or left ventricular hypertrophy. If an arrhythmia is suspected but not identified on an ECG trace, you may consider arranging a 24-hour ECG recording. Lying and standing blood pressure recordings will show whether orthostatic hypotension is present. A chest X-ray can show calcified cardiac valves, cardiac enlargement and pulmonary oedema, pointing to a cardiac cause for the collapse. In this instance, an echocardiogram will quantify the degree of the aortic stenosis.

Medical therapy, such as diuretics, can offer some benefit; but ultimately, patients require an interventional procedure to improve aortic valve function. Ideally, an aortic valve replacement will be carried out. Patients should be reviewed by a cardiologist, who can judge the best time for the procedure to be carried out – usually when the patient develops significant symptoms. In frail patients who may not be able to tolerate an aortic valve replacement, a transcatheter aortic valve implantation (TAVI), which is comparatively less invasive, improves morbidity and mortality.

KEY POINTS

- In a patient who has transiently lost consciousness, a broad differential diagnosis should be considered. Possible causes include cardiac arrhythmias, cardiac obstruction, orthostatic hypotension and epileptic seizures.
- An eye-witness account is very helpful in identifying the possible cause of loss of consciousness.
- Aortic stenosis can cause symptoms of fatigue, angina and collapse. When a patient develops these symptoms, an aortic valve replacement will ideally be carried out. In frail patients, a transcatheter aortic valve implantation may be a more suitable option.

CASE 28: PALPITATIONS AND COLLAPSE

History
A 24-year-old man was in a pub when he suddenly collapsed. When the paramedics arrived he had come around and an ECG was performed (Fig. 28.1). He described feeling palpitations prior to his collapse and has had this before. He was feeling unwell, cool and clammy. His blood pressure was 101/72 mmHg. He was taken to the emergency department.

Examination
This young man became more unwell and drowsy. His blood pressure on arrival was 60/40 mmHg. A new ECG was performed (Fig. 28.2).

Initial treatment
He underwent urgent synchronized DC cardioversion which restored him to sinus rhythm. Cardiovascular and respiratory examination was normal. He was taken to the coronary care unit for monitoring.

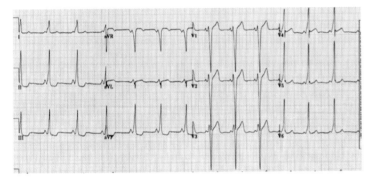

Figure 28.1

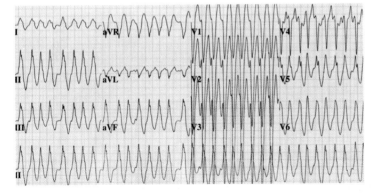

Figure 28.2

Questions
- What is the underlying diagnosis?
- What caused this patient to decompensate?
- How should he be managed?

ANSWER 28

Figure 28.1 demonstrates a short PR interval with a slurred onset of the QRS waveform (delta wave). When associated with a supraventricular tachycardia the diagnosis is Wolff–Parkinson–White (WPW) syndrome. The cause of the delta wave is due to an accessory conduction pathway that is separate from the usual AV node/bundle of His–Purkinje conduction pathway. The extra pathway connects the atria to the ventricles. During sinus rhythm the SA node activates both conduction pathways, resulting in depolarization of the ventricles from two separate places. As a result the PR interval is shortened and there is a slurred upstroke (delta wave) at the beginning of ventricular depolarization. The delta wave is seen in sinus rhythm and not during tachycardias associated with WPW. Sometimes the pathway is 'concealed'; i.e. there is no short PR interval and slurred upstroke as there is no antegrade conduction. A tachycardia can result if a re-entry circuit is set up involving the accessory pathway and the normal AV nodal pathway. As there is no AV node in the accessory pathway to limit atrial conduction, ventricular rates can be very fast. This has the potential to cause syncope, haemodynamic compromise or sudden death. However, sudden death is rare (estimated frequency of 0.1 per cent).

In the presence of atrial fibrillation the re-entry tachycardia can be potentially fatal. Very fast fibrillation causes rapidly conducted rates of above 220/min which can trigger ventricular fibrillation. This occurrence is quite rare. In this case his rhythm has changed to atrial fibrillation with rapid conduction to the ventricles causing him to decompensate.

The immediate management in anyone with unstable tachycardia is urgent synchronized DC cardioversion. If the patient is haemodynamically stable but the ECG demonstrates a regular tachycardia, then AV node blocking medications can be used. If this does not work, electrical cardioversion is used. If the underlying rhythm is AF, avoidance of AV blocking drugs like digoxin, adenosine, calcium-channel antagonists and beta-blockers is important. Intravenous amiodarone or procainamide can be used as these drugs prolong the refractory period of the accessory pathway. Again, electrical cardioversion is required if there is no response to medications. An echocardiogram should be performed to rule out structural heart abnormalities that are associated with accessory pathways (Ebstein's anomaly and hypertrophic cardiomyopathy). Long-term management will require referral to an electrophysiologist to consider ablation of the pathway.

 KEY POINTS

- An ECG with a short PR interval and delta wave describes the WPW pattern – its association with palpitations and SVT describes the syndrome. However, the WPW pattern is absent in concealed pathways.
- WPW syndrome is associated with sudden death but the incidence of this is extremely rare.

CASE 29: ECCHYMOSIS

History
A 31-year-old woman has presented to the emergency department with significant bruising on her arms and legs that has been getting worse. She first noticed them five days ago when they started off as small bruises. She intended to visit her GP but noticed they were now larger and more widespread. She has had no fevers, arthralgia or recent viral infections, and she is not taking any medications.

Examination
This woman looks systemically well. There is a marked petechial rash over her legs with large bruising on the arms and legs. A cardiovascular and respiratory exam is normal. On abdominal examination there is no hepatosplenomegaly and there is no lymphadenopathy. Observations: temperature 36.8°C, heart rate 78/min, blood pressure 135/67 mmHg, respiratory rate 18/min, SaO_2 98 per cent on air.

INVESTIGATIONS		
		Normal range
White cells	6.0	$4–11 \times 10^9/L$
Haemoglobin	11.1	13–18 g/dL
Platelets	15	$150–400 \times 10^9/L$
Sodium	133	135–145 mmol/L
Potassium	3.7	3.5–5.0 mmol/L
Urea	5.4	3.0–7.0 mmol/L
Creatinine	65	60–110 µmol/L
INR	1.0	0.9–1.1
APTT	23	18–28 s
Blood film	Reduced platelet count, no abnormal white cells	

Questions
- What is the most likely diagnosis?
- How should this patient be managed?

ANSWER 29

The main abnormality in the results is the very low platelet count. The most likely diagnosis is idiopathic thrombocytopenic purpura (ITP). However, she requires other investigations to exclude causes such as B_{12} or folate deficiency, acute leukaemia or sepsis. An abdominal ultrasound should be performed to check the size of the spleen and look for any other masses as an enlarged spleen indicates an alternative diagnosis. An HIV test is also advised. Bone marrow aspirate and biopsy can determine whether platelet production is normal and hence the likely cause of low platelets is immune-mediated antibody destruction in the spleen. In general a bone marrow biopsy is not required in a young, systemically well person but would be considered if there were other features suggesting an alternative diagnosis or failure to respond to treatment. In the absence of medications and infective causes, ITP is the likely cause.

Her bruising is worsening and, based on her history, examination, platelet count and blood film, ITP should be treated with intravenous immunoglobulin and prednisolone. If there is life-threatening bleeding, such as an intracranial bleed, platelet transfusion in addition to immunoglobulin/steroid therapy can be given. Tranexamic acid can also be administered as this helps to inhibit fibrinolysis and stabilize clot formation.

If bleeding is uncontrolled despite therapy, a splenectomy can be performed.

 KEY POINTS

- Idiopathic thrombocytopenic purpura is a diagnosis of exclusion and there is no confirmatory test for it.
- If the spleen is enlarged then another cause is more likely, such as systemic lupus erythematosus (SLE).

History

A 49-year-old woman suddenly developed right arm and leg weakness and has been brought to the emergency department. She describes a one-week history of feeling tired and weak, with some confusion. Her medical history includes hypertension, hypercholesterolaemia and hypothyroidism. She is taking ramipril, simvastatin and levothyroxine. She does not smoke and drinks wine only occasionally.

Examination

This woman has petechiae over her legs. Cardiovascular, respiratory and abdominal exams are normal. Neurological exam shows mild weakness of the arm and leg but no sensation disturbance or visual disturbance. No higher cortical dysfunction is found. A CT head scan does not show any bleeding. Observations: temperature 37.8°C, heart rate 76/min, blood pressure 154/89 mmHg, respiratory rate 16/min, SaO_2 96 per cent on air.

INVESTIGATIONS		
		Normal range
White cells	9.0	$4–11 \times 10^9$/L
Haemoglobin	7.1	13–18 g/dL
Reticulocytes	5	0.5–1% of RBC
Platelets	12	$150–400 \times 10^9$/L
Sodium	140	135–145 mmol/L
Potassium	5.1	3.5–5.0 mmol/L
Urea	24.2	3.0–7.0 mmol/L
Creatinine	195	60–110 µmol/L
Blood film	Schistocytes and low platelet count	
Direct Coombs test	Negative	

Questions
- What is the most likely diagnosis?
- How would you manage this patient?

ANSWER 30

This patient has anaemia, thrombocytopenia, red cell fragments on blood film, normal clotting profile with petechiae, fever, neurological signs and impaired renal function. These findings are consistent with thrombotic thrombocytopenic purpura (TTP). The classic description is a pentad of microangiopathic haemolytic anaemia, thrombocytopenic purpura, neurological dysfunction, renal dysfunction and fever. However, most cases of TTP do not have all five features.

TTP is caused by large von Willebrand factor multimers which form platelet aggregates that cause microvascular thrombosis in organs such as the brain and kidneys. Normally von Willebrand factor is cleaved by ADAMTS-13 to prevent large multimers forming. In TTP an autoimmune reaction is thought to deplete ADAMTS-13. The cause of this is not clear.

Differential diagnoses include haemolytic uraemic syndrome associated with *E. coli* 0157:H7 infection, disseminated intravascular coagulation (DIC: would get a prolonged PT and APTT with elevated D-dimers) and malignant hypertension (BP >200 mmHg systolic and >130 mmHg diastolic).

Untreated TTP is fatal and she presents with neurological and renal dysfunction. Immediate management should be to arrange plasma exchange within 24 hours of presentation. She should also be started on corticosteroids. The duration of plasma exchange can be gauged by the response in platelet count and reduction in LDH level. If there is active bleeding, platelet transfusion and blood can be given. There is some uncertainty as to the role of antiplatelet agents in the acute setting to prevent platelet aggregation; however, due to low platelet counts their use is controversial.

 KEY POINTS

- Plasma exchange is the mainstay of treatment in thrombotic thrombocytopenic purpura. When started early it can reduce mortality to between 10 and 30 per cent.
- TTP presents with neurological signs in about half of cases.
- The pathophysiology is similar to HUS. Please refer to Case 18 (p. 35).

CASE 31: GENERALIZED WEAKNESS AND DYSARTHRIA

History

A 74-year-old man has presented to the emergency department complaining of generalized progressive weakness to the point that he cannot get up from a chair. This had been getting worse over a period of six months. Initially he had weakness from rising up from sitting or on walking up stairs. He has also noticed a dry mouth, loss of weight and cough over the last few months. He has a history of mild chronic obstructive pulmonary disease (COPD) and is a former smoker of 50 pack years. He does not drink alcohol. He takes calcium supplementation and a tiotropium inhaler. He feels dizzy on standing.

Examination

On neurological testing he is found to have generalized weakness, more marked proximally than distally. His tendon reflexes are reduced. His speech is noted to be dysarthric and he has diplopia and ptosis. Cardiovascular, respiratory and abdominal examinations are unremarkable. Blood pressure is 134/89 mmHg sitting and 121/74 mmHg standing. A chest X-ray shows a spiculated mass in the right upper lobe and hilar lymphadenopathy.

Questions

- What is the most likely cause of this man's neurological symptoms?
- How is this condition diagnosed?
- What would be the appropriate management?

ANSWER 31

This patient has a progressive neuromuscular condition characterized by weakness more marked in proximal muscles and reduced tendon reflexes. Other features are dysarthria, diplopia and ptosis which occur in myasthenia gravis. He also has autonomic features (dry mouth and postural hypotension). These are characteristic of Lambert–Eaton myasthenic syndrome (LEMS). Malignancy is associated with half of LEMS cases. Small-cell lung cancer is the most commonly associated underlying malignancy. This patient has an abnormal chest X-ray and a CT chest with tissue diagnosis is required.

LEMS is diagnosed with nerve conduction studies, which show an incremental muscle response to repeated electrical stimulation. Auto-antibodies to voltage-gated calcium channels (VGCC) are associated with LEMS that is not associated with cancer. In these cases other autoimmune conditions can be associated with it.

This man has generalized weakness and, although dysarthric, he has no bulbar weakness and no evidence of respiratory compromise. If he were to develop these complications he may require intubation and respiratory support. In this case treatment is for his lung cancer as this is likely to improve symptoms. He should receive thromboprophylaxis and avoid drugs that impair neuromuscular transmission (calcium-channel blockers, lithium, magnesium). Amifampridine is a drug that may be used to increase neuromuscular transmission. Its use should be in consultation with a specialist.

In other cases of LEMS that do not respond to drugs that increase neuromuscular transmission, prednisolone with or without azathioprine is used. Some may even require plasma exchange or intravenous immunoglobulin treatment.

 KEY POINTS

- Lambert–Eaton myasthenic syndrome is strongly associated with malignancy (50 per cent of cases), so patients presenting with symptoms of LEMS should undergo appropriate screening.
- LEMS is diagnosed with nerve conduction studies, which show an incremental muscle response to repeated electrical stimulation.

CASE 32: DYSPHAGIA AND SHALLOW BREATHING

History

A 32-year-old woman has presented to the emergency department with increasing difficulty in swallowing and difficulty in breathing. She is also unable to lift her arms and her head keeps drooping. These symptoms appeared after a recent chest infection. Last year she had visited her GP because of double vision that worsened with reading and with intermittent weakness. She also noted difficulty in talking after prolonged speech. However, symptoms were mild and occasional only and no treatment was required. She has no medical history, is not on medications and is generally fit and well.

Examination

This woman looks fatigued and has droopy eyelids. She breathes quickly and shallowly. A neurological examination reveales proximal muscle weakness and bilateral mild ptosis but no muscle wasting or abnormal reflexes. The rest of the cardiovascular, respiratory and abdominal examination is unremarkable. Observations: blood pressure 127/62 mmHg, heart rate 62/min, respiratory rate 28/min.

Questions
- What is the most likely diagnosis?
- How would you manage this patient?

ANSWER 32

This woman has dysphagia, respiratory distress and generalized weakness. In the context of earlier intermittent symptoms of fatiguable muscular weakness affecting speech and vision, she is likely to suffer from myasthenia gravis and now presents in a myasthenic crisis. A crisis is often provoked within the first two years of diagnosis and is precipitated by infections, aspiration or drugs.

Myasthenia gravis (MG) is a chronic autoimmune disorder affecting the neuromuscular junction of skeletal muscles. Antibodies against the nicotinic acetylcholine receptor cause destruction of the post-synaptic membrane. Hence skeletal muscle weakness occurs. MG can affect just the ocular muscles or also can involve other muscle groups such as limb and axial muscles or oropharyngeal and respiratory muscles. Muscle weakness can be graded as mild to severe. Severe muscle weakness of the oropharyngeal and respiratory groups can compromise the airway. Infection can worsen MG.

Tests to confirm MG include serum anti-acetylcholine receptor antibody; if this is negative, anti-muscle tyrosine kinase antibody is commonly present. If antibodies are negative, repetitive nerve testing can be performed to demonstrate a successive decrement in action potentials. A CT chest is performed in newly diagnosed cases to rule out an associated thymoma. The major differential is LEMS; however, in this case the history points towards MG and there are no autonomic features. LEMS is also usually associated with an underlying malignancy or with anti-VGCC antibodies in those without cancer. Other myopathies can present with muscle weakness, but they are not fatiguable – which is characteristic of MG.

This woman has a myasthenic crisis precipitated by pneumonia and is at risk of respiratory failure. Her forced vital capacity (FVC) should be measured: an FVC of 15 mL/kg or less would suggest the need for mechanical ventilator support. To reverse the process she will need either intravenous immunoglobulin or plasma exchange. Even if she does not require intubation she should be closely monitored by serial FVC and treated in an intensive-care setting where intubation can be performed.

Once she has responded to acute treatment, pyridostigmine is required in the long term. Some patients with severe MG require regular intermittent intravenous immunoglobulin therapy every month. Other immunosuppressant therapy (e.g. prednisolone, azathioprine, ciclosporin) may be needed for maintenance treatment.

 KEY POINTS

- Myasthenia crisis can be precipitated by infection, aspiration, trauma, drugs, surgery or pregnancy.
- Myasthenia gravis presenting with oropharyngeal weakness or shortness of breath should alert you to potential respiratory compromise.

History

A 72-year-old man has presented to his GP after noticing large blisters developing over his arms, legs and lower abdomen. Some have burst and are uncomfortable. This condition started about five days ago. He is otherwise completely well, although he relates that he has had itchy skin for the last couple of months. He is not on any medications.

Examination

There were tense blisters mostly over the arms and legs but involving the groin and abdomen. Some of the blisters appear clear but others are bloodstained. A few blisters have burst, leaving an erythematous, moist base. His mouth shows no abnormalities. A cardiorespiratory and abdominal examination is normal. Observations: temperature 37.1°C, blood pressure 146/72 mmHg, heart rate 74/min, respiratory rate 15/min, SaO_2 100 per cent on room air.

Questions
- What is the most likely diagnosis?
- How would you further investigate and manage this patient?

ANSWER 34

The symptoms and signs are consistent with a tension pneumothorax: reduced air entry, resonance to percussion, and deviation of the mediastinum to the other side.

Tension develops when air accumulates during inspiration and is not released during expiration. This situation can result from disruption of the pleura and surrounding tissue so that a one-way valve is created, resulting in air only flowing in and not out. With each breath this causes a progressive build-up of air and thus pressure within the pleural cavity, resulting in compression of the lung tissue and surrounding mediastinal structures. It is thought that blood flow to the heart becomes restricted from compression to the superior vena cava as well as compressing the atria and ultimately the ventricle causing tamponade. Cardiac output falls and cardiogenic shock ensues. Tracheal deviation is therefore a relatively late sign. Hypotension is an ominous sign.

This is a medical emergency and immediate decompression is required. Decompression is achieved by inserting a 14-gauge cannula into the pleural space at the second intercostal space and midclavicular line. Enough trapped air can then escape through the cannula to relieve the positive pressure in the chest and allow cardiac filling with improved cardiac output. Meanwhile a chest drain should be inserted.

The diagnosis of a tension pneumothorax is based on a clinical examination, and treatment should be started before a chest X-ray is arranged. A tension pneumothorax can occur with any type of pneumothorax, whether the cause is spontaneous, secondary to underlying pulmonary disease, or caused by traumatic injury from blunt or penetrating injury to the chest wall. In this scenario what makes a tension pneumothorax most likely is the rapidity of the onset of signs with worsening chest pain. The diagnosis can, however, be less clear-cut and present with a more insidious course until the patient is in extremis.

This patient's chest X-ray shows a large right-sided pneumothorax with some mediastinal deviation. As mentioned above, treatment of a tension pneumothorax should be immediate, so a chest X-ray like this should never be obtained! In this case, the patient required a chest drain to be inserted for 48 hours, and the lung gradually re-expanded. She was advised to avoid contact sport for six weeks and that she should never dive, as a pneumothorax while diving could be fatal.

 KEY POINTS

- Tension pneumothorax, although rare, is a medical emergency. Immediate recognition of signs and urgent needle decompression is required. Do not wait for a chest X-ray.
- Any cause of pneumothorax can result in a tension pneumothorax.

History

A 63-year-old man has visited his GP with progressive swelling of his legs over a period of a month. He has also noticed that his urine is more frothy than usual. He does not complain of cough, shortness of breath or chest pains. There is no loss of weight or fever. He has no significant medical history. He drinks wine on occasion, does not smoke and is not on any medications. He is a retired painter and decorator.

Examination

This man has pitting oedema up to the thighs. His blood pressure is 135/80 mmHg, pulse 72/min and regular, and respiratory rate 12/min. A cardiovascular, respiratory, abdominal and neurological examination is normal.

INVESTIGATIONS		
		Normal range
White cells	8.0	$4–11 \times 10^9$/L
Haemoglobin	15.0	13–18 g/dL
Platelets	350	$150–400 \times 10^9$/L
Sodium	128	135–145 mmol/L
Potassium	3.7	3.5–5.0 mmol/L
Urea	5.8	3.0–7.0 mmol/L
Creatinine	86	60–110 µmol/L
Bilirubin	8	5–25 µmol/L
Alanine aminotransferase	30	8–55 IU/L
Alkaline phosphatase	52	42–98 IU/L
Albumin	21	35–50 g/L
Urinalysis	Protein ++++, no blood	
24-hour urinary protein	11 g	

Questions

- What is the most likely diagnosis?
- How should the patient be further investigated and managed?

ANSWER 35

The presence of oedema, hypoalbuminaemia (<30 g/L) and significant proteinuria (>3.5 g in 24 hours) are diagnostic of nephrotic syndrome. In particular this man does not have another cause for oedema (e.g. cardiac failure) or other cause of hypoalbuminaemia (protein-losing enteropathy or chronic liver disease). This condition is also associated with hyperlipidaemia and a hypercoagulable state.

It is important to establish a quick diagnosis of nephrotic syndrome. A spot urine protein:creatinine test is increasingly replacing 24-hour collections (>3.5 g in 24 hours is equivalent to a protein:creatinine ratio [PCR] of >200 mg/μmol).

Nephrotic syndrome, however, is a collection of features that are caused by an underlying disease process. The disease is targeted at the glomerular basement membrane. Proteins are normally prevented from passing through the membrane by a network of connections between the foot processes of podocytes. If this barrier is disrupted then proteins leak out. A lack of albumin in the plasma results in reduced oncotic pressure, causing water to leak out into the interstitial tissue. Clotting factors, immunoglobulins and complement also pass through the defective membrane.

The disease processes that result in nephrotic syndrome are:

- primary glomerular disease: minimal change disease, focal segmental glomerulosclerosis, membranous nephropathy;
- systemic disease: diabetic nephropathy, multiple myeloma, IgA nephropathy, SLE, amyloidosis;
- infections: HBV, HCV, HIV, post-streptococcal, syphilis, endocarditis;
- malignancy: Hodgkin's lymphoma and other solid organ tumours;
- drugs: gold, penicillamine, NSAIDs, captopril, lithium;
- other rare causes: Alport's syndrome, Fabry's disease, nail–patella syndrome.

Since the list of causes is long, a thorough history and examination is essential.

The most common cause of nephrotic syndrome in the elderly is membranous nephropathy; underlying malignancy is the most common cause of secondary membranous nephropathy.

Investigations should be guided by the history and examination findings. The cause of nephrotic syndrome in adults often requires a renal biopsy for a definitive diagnosis. Therefore anyone presenting with features of nephrotic syndrome should be referred to a renal specialist.

It is generally recommended that inpatients should be on prophylactic heparin to prevent venous thromboembolism secondary to the hypercoagulable state. There is a potential to develop arterial and venous thromboses. In particular, renal vein thromboses can occur and this should be suspected if there is a rapid deterioration in renal function with or without flank pain or haematuria.

In this case, the patient was found to have type 2 diabetes mellitus, which caused a membranous nephropathy. A renal biopsy was required to make the diagnosis. Following supportive treatment with fluid restriction and renal function monitoring, as well as improving the patient's blood glucose and cholesterol levels, he made a good recovery.

KEY POINTS

- Nephrotic syndrome is associated with infections, venous and arterial thromboses and dyslipidaemia.
- Nephrotic syndrome in adults often requires a renal biopsy to determine the underlying cause.

History
A 60-year-old man has presented to the emergency department with a two-week history of haemoptysis, dry cough and shortness of breath. He has also noticed that his urine has become darker. He came back from Spain four weeks ago and has felt non-specifically unwell since. He smokes 15 cigarettes per day and drinks 4 pints of beer per week. He is on no medications. He works as a lorry driver.

Examination
This man has bibasal inspiratory crackles on auscultation of the chest. The rest of the cardiorespiratory, abdominal and neurological examination is normal. A chest X-ray shows bilateral patchy shadowing in the lower zones. Observations: blood pressure 165/85 mmHg, heart rate 85/min, respiratory rate 24/min, SaO_2 92 per cent on room air.

INVESTIGATIONS		
		Normal range
White cells	9.2	$4–11 \times 10^9$/L
Haemoglobin	11.0	13–18 g/dL
Mean cell volume	76	82–100 fL
Platelets	450	$150–400 \times 10^9$/L
Sodium	138	135–145 mmol/L
Potassium	5.0	3.5–5.0 mmol/L
Urea	19	3.0–7.0 mmol/L
Creatinine	280	60–110 µmol/L
INR	1.2	0.9–1.1
Urine dipstick	Blood +++	
Urine microscopy	Red cell casts	

Questions
- What is the likely diagnosis and how can you confirm this?
- How would you manage this patient?

ANSWER 36

This man has a pulmonary–renal syndrome, specifically glomerulonephritis and pulmonary haemorrhage, and the most likely diagnosis is Goodpasture's syndrome. There are other causes of pulmonary renal syndromes and a definitive diagnosis relies on testing for anti-glomerular basement membrane antibody titre and a renal biopsy which will show crescentic glomerulonephritis and linear IgG staining. An ANCA (antineutrophil cytoplasmic antibodies) test should be performed to rule out Wegener's granulomatosis, Churg–Strauss syndrome and microscopic polyarteritis. In 30–50 per cent of cases those with Goodpasture's syndrome will also test positive for ANCA. Antinuclear antibody (ANA) and serum complement C3 and C4 are useful to exclude lupus nephritis.

Goodpasture's syndrome, or anti-glomerular basement membrane (GBM) disease, is caused by an auto-antibody to type 4 collagen, which is present in the lung and the glomerular basement membrane. The cause of the disease is not certain, but there is an association with smoking. A genetic predisposition has also been suggested.

Immediate management should focus on ensuring he is receiving adequate oxygenation. If pulmonary haemorrhage is severe he may need further respiratory support such as intubation. He is currently haemodynamically stable and has a normal clotting profile. He has pulmonary haemorrhage which is potentially fatal. A renal opinion should be sought as a matter of urgency to establish a diagnosis with a renal biopsy. This will enable appropriate treatment.

First-line therapy involves pulsed methylprednisolone (1 g intravenously for three days) followed by prednisolone (1 mg/kg/day orally, maximum dose 80 mg/day). Plasma exchange and cyclophosphamide are also used. Even those who test positive for ANCA are initially treated in the same manner, but longer term cyclophosphamide and prednisolone are required. If renal impairment is severe enough to require haemodialysis, there is usually a low likelihood of renal recovery.

A full blood count needs to be monitored weekly while on cyclophosphamide as this can cause leucopenia. Renal impairment does not always fully resolve and chronic kidney disease may occur. Cigarette smoking is strongly discouraged.

 KEY POINTS

- Recognition of a pulmonary–renal syndrome with early diagnosis and treatment offers the best chance of renal function recovery.
- Pulmonary haemorrhage is potentially fatal and requires urgent treatment with corticosteroids, plasma exhange and cyclophosphamide.
- It is relatively common to have both anti-GBM and ANCA antibodies.

CASE 37: KNEE SWELLING AND PAIN

History

A 75-year-old man has presented to the emergency department with severe pain in his knee. This started two days ago and he is now unable to walk. He has a history of hypertension and heart failure for which he has been taking lisinopril, bisoprolol, aspirin, simvastatin and bendroflumethiazide. Recently furosemide was added to his treatment because of increasing ankle oedema.

Examination

This elderly man's left knee is swollen with evidence of an effusion, and it is erythematous and tender to the touch and painful on any movement. No other joints are affected. There is no skin rash. A sample of fluid aspirated from the knee is initially bloodstained; then straw-coloured turbid fluid is obtained. Observations: temperature 37.9°C, blood pressure 142/86 mmHg, heart rate of 76/min, respiratory rate 18/min. A knee X-ray reveals no bony abnormalities.

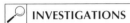

INVESTIGATIONS	
Synovial fluid:	
White cells	18 000/mL (75% neutrophils)
No organisms seen	
Negatively birefringent crystals seen	

Questions

- What is the most likely diagnosis?
- What is the most important differential diagnosis?
- How would you manage this patient?

This man has gout. This is characterized by an acute onset of pain and swelling of a joint. Synovial fluid microscopy demonstrates crystals that under polarized light are negatively birefringent.

Gout is a condition in which urate crystals deposit within joints causing an inflammatory arthritis. They can also deposit in the glomerulus and cause tubular and interstitial disease as well as uric acid stones. Gout occurs more commonly in men and increases in incidence with age. Gout is associated with hyperuricaemia, although elevated levels of uric acid do not always result in gout. Risk factors for gout include old age, male sex, medications such as thiazide and loop diuretics and aspirin. Some people have tophi from urate deposits on hands, the helix of the ears or over extensor surfaces.

The most important diagnosis to exclude is septic arthritis. Diagnosis is based on synovial fluid microscopy and culture. The patient may also present with systemic signs of sepsis.

The other main differential is pseudogout. That presents in exactly the same way as an acute attack of gout except that the cause is calcium pyrophosphate crystals which are only weakly positively birefringent rhomboid-shaped crystals. Chondrocalcinosis may also be seen on X-ray. Other possible diagnoses include rheumatoid arthritis, reactive arthritis and psoriatic arthritis.

Initially, non-steroidal anti-inflammatory drugs (NSAIDs) such as naproxen, ibuprofen or diclofenac provide symptom relief and anti-inflammatory benefits. If there are contra-indications to NSAIDs (e.g. GI bleed from a peptic ulcer), colchicine is an alternative. Side-effects are common and include diarrhoea, nausea and vomiting. An intra-articular injection of corticosteroid can be used or a short course of oral prednisolone (20–40 mg once daily for one week). To prevent recurrent episodes, the xanthine oxidase inhibitor allopurinol can be started when the acute phase has settled.

In a few cases, very high uric acid levels can precipitate nephropathy and renal failure. This can occur in conditions of tumour lysis such as when patients are treated with cyto-toxic chemotherapy for malignancies.

KEY POINTS

- Gout is a condition in which urate crystals deposit within joints causing an inflammatory arthritis.
- Gout can have a similar presentation to pseudogout. They can be differentiated by looking at the synovial fluid under a microscope. In gout there are negatively birefringent crystals, whereas in pseudogout there are positively birefringent rhomboid-shaped crystals.
- Urate crystals may be deposited in the glomeruli and lead to tubular and interstitial disease as well as uric acid stones. High urate levels can also cause a nephropathy and eventually renal failure.

History

A 62-year-old man has presented to the emergency department following a large rectal bleed. He has been experiencing intermittent episodes of bleeding over the last few months. He describes them as sometimes dark and sometimes bright red and not confined to bowel movements. There is no abdominal pain, change in bowel habit or loss of weight. He has no previous significant medical history. He does not take any regular medications and does not drink alcohol. There is no family medical history of significance. He works as a plumber.

Examination

On rectal examination there is fresh blood but no peri-anal lesions. The rest of the gastrointestinal examination is normal. On cardiovascular examination there is a harsh ejection systolic murmur, but respiratory examination is unremarkable. He is afebrile. Observations: blood pressure 95/65 mmHg, heart rate 102/min, respiratory rate 18/min, SaO_2 95 per cent on room air.

INVESTIGATIONS		
		Normal range
White cells	6.7	$4–11 \times 10^9/L$
Haemoglobin	8.1	13–18 g/dL
Platelets	220	$150–400 \times 10^9/L$
Sodium	138	135–145 mmol/L
Potassium	3.8	3.5–5.0 mmol/L
Urea	4.0	3.0–7.0 mmol/L
Creatinine	82	60–110 µmol/L
INR	1.0	0.9–1.1

Questions
- What further investigations would be appropriate?
- What is the probable diagnosis?
- How would you manage this patient immediately and in the longer term?

ANSWER 38

This patient has an acute gastrointestinal (GI) bleed. It is likely this is lower GI in origin because of the fresh blood on rectal examination, but a brisk upper GI bleed could also present in this way.

Immediate management involves obtaining haemodynamic stability. He is hypotensive, tachycardic with evidence of ongoing bleeding. He therefore requires resuscitation with intravenous fluids – preferably blood. This can be obtained in an emergency setting as group O negative. While waiting for this, colloid or crystalloid fluids should be administered. He should have two large-bore cannulae sited peripherally and bloods taken for urgent cross-matching.

If the bleeding continues and he remains haemodynamically unstable, he should initially undergo an upper GI endoscopy to rule out a proximal cause. If this does not identify the cause and there is active bleeding, a mesenteric angiogram can identify the source of bleeding. At the same time the radiologist can carry out embolization of the feeder vessel. Colonoscopy or surgery may be required if mesenteric angiography is unavailable or does not stop the bleeding.

Regular full blood count, clotting profile with fibrinogen levels should be undertaken to ensure haemoglobin, platelets and clotting factors are optimally replaced.

In this case the history might be in keeping with angiodysplasia, but an urgent oesophago-gastro-duodenoscopy (OGD) and/or colonoscopy may help to ascertain the underlying cause. Angiodysplasia is a condition where the small vessels in the bowel are dilated, very fragile and prone to bleeding. Areas of angiodsyplasia can occur throughout the entire GI tract but are most common in the ascending colon. This patient's history also indicates the presence of possible aortic stenosis. In some case series there is an association with colonic angiodysplasia but this is not certain. Often in this situation where the patient is unstable, investigation forms part of treatment and the goal is to stop bleeding and resuscitate. If his bleeding were to stop spontaneously and resuscitation was successful, an elective colonoscopy would then be the most appropriate test. If no source of bleeding is found, an OGD should be performed. Bleeding secondary to angiodysplasia normally stops spontaneously in the majority of patients. There is a risk of rebleeding: rates up to 15 per cent at two years after an untreated colonic bleed. Poor prognosis is associated with shock at presentation, the presence of co-morbidities, and the requirement for emergency surgery.

An acute lower GI bleed is defined as bleeding from the GI tract distal to the ligament of Treitz at the junction between the fourth part of the duodenum and proximal jejunum. Lower GI bleeds represent 20 per cent of all cases of acute GI haemorrhage. The most common causes are diverticular disease and angiodysplasia.

 KEY POINTS

- The passage of fresh red blood per rectum can be a result of upper or lower GI bleeding.
- Initial management should be resuscitation followed by an OGD.
- Angiodysplasia of the colon is the second most common cause of GI bleeding in patients over the age of 60 years (diverticular disease being the most common in that age group). The most common presentation is intermittent bleeding without pain.

CASE 39: SHORTNESS OF BREATH AND PEDAL OEDEMA

History

A 52-year-old man presented to the emergency department because of progressive dyspnoea over four weeks. Prior to this he was completely well. He had no history of heart disease, lung problems or diabetes. He has been told he has high blood pressure but is not receiving any treatment for it. He smokes 10 cigarettes per day and drinks about 4 pints of lager per week.

Examination

The man was noted to be overweight. His jugular venous pulse was elevated. Heart sounds were normal, but there were bibasal inspiratory crackles in the chest, and pedal oedema. Observations: temperature 36.5°C, blood pressure 164/84 mmHg, heart rate 150/min, respiratory rate 22/min, SaO_2 96 per cent on room air.

A chest X-ray showed small bilateral pleural effusions and cardiomegaly. An ECG was performed (Fig. 39.1).

Initial treatment

In the emergency department he was given adenosine, and his heart rate slowed to 70 beats per minute. The following day he had a further episode of tachycardia and was therefore loaded with digoxin. Twenty-four hours later his heart rate settled to 70 beats per minute. An echocardiogram was performed which showed moderately impaired LV function. He was commenced on a diuretic and a beta-blocker and ACE-inhibitor were started.

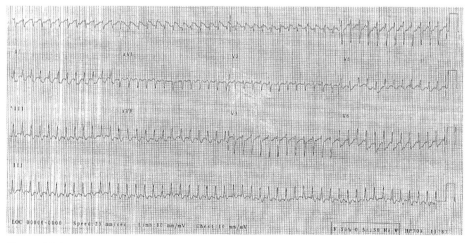

Figure 39.1

Questions

- What is the diagnosis?
- How would you manage this patient?

ANSWER 39

The ECG shows a regular rate at almost 300/min but it is difficult to make out the P waves. It is likely that this is atrial flutter with 1:1 conduction, as his subsequent ECG shows atrial flutter. Differential diagnoses of a supraventricular tachycardia (SVT) include sinus tachycardia, atrial fibrillation and flutter, AV nodal re-entry tachycardia, AV re-entry tachycardia and multifocal atrial tachycardia.

In this case adenosine was administered to block the AV node conduction transiently. This allows dissociation of atrial and ventricular activity, which can either treat the underlying cause or help diagnose the underlying rhythm abnormality. In atrial fibrillation and flutter the atria continue to depolarize but the conduction to the ventricles is halted for a brief period. An ECG strip will show either an irregular baseline of disorganized P-wave activity or the sawtooth appearance of regular p-wave activity at 300/min in atrial flutter. AV nodal re-entry tachycardia can be terminated with adenosine as it blocks the re-entry circuit that involves the AV node itself.

Management of any SVT depends on the condition of the patient. If the patient shows signs of shock, heart failure or myocardial ischaemia then he/she should be electrically cardioverted with a synchronized DC shock. If the patient is stable, the underlying rhythm should be determined to guide treatment. For regular SVT, as in this case, adenosine is the drug of first choice. This may well terminate the tachycardia. If flutter is the underlying rhythm then rate control is the aim (e.g. beta-blocker or digoxin). In this case the man had features of mild fluid overload but was haemodynamically stable, so digoxin was commenced. Fast irregular rates are likely to be atrial fibrillation, and then rate control is the initial treatment of choice.

It is important to perform an echocardiogram to determine any underlying cause for the rhythm disturbance. Fast atrial fibrillation or flutter of several weeks' duration can lead to a rate-related cardiomyopathy which improves with rate control. A repeat echocardiogram is needed once the rate is controlled to see whether LV function has improved.

 KEY POINTS

- Atrial flutter as well as fibrillation increases the risk of stroke. Anticoagulation should be considered.
- Supraventricular tachycardia has various causes.
- Immediate treatment is dependent on patient stability. Unstable patients require immediate electrical cardioversion.

CASE 40: SHARP CENTRAL CHEST PAIN

History

A 42-year-old woman has presented to the emergency department with chest pain. It is central, sharp in nature, and made worse by inspiration and by lying down. The pain eases when she sits forward. She had no medical history and is taking no medications. She is a non-smoker and does not drink alcohol. She works as a healthcare assistant.

Examination

On examination of the precordium there is a rub heard at the left lower sternal edge in systole and diastole. The rest of the cardiorespiratory and abdominal examination is unremarkable. Observations: temperature 37.6°C, heart rate 98/min, blood pressure 121/72 mmHg, respiratory rate 18/min, SaO_2 100 per cent on room air.

A chest X-ray shows a normal-sized heart and clear lung fields. An ECG shows widespread ST elevation (Fig. 40.1).

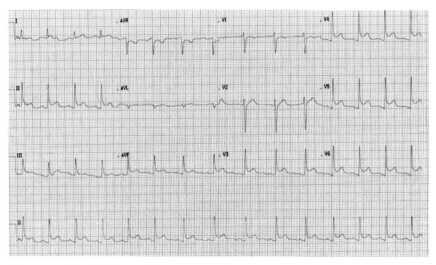

Figure 40.1 Supplied by Dr Stam Kapetanakis

Questions

- What is the most likely diagnosis?
- How would you manage this patient?

ANSWER 40

This patient's signs and symptoms with the ECG changes are consistent with an acute pericarditis. Viral pericarditis is the most common cause and is associated with coxsackievirus B and influenza epidemics. Other causes include autoimmune diseases and uraemia associated with renal failure.

She should have an echocardiogram, which is usually normal but sometimes shows evidence of a pericardial effusion, which may need to be monitored. A large pericardial effusion can cause cardiac tamponade, and a pericardiocentesis is sometimes required to drain off the fluid.

It is likely that this woman has a viral pericarditis, which is usually a limiting disease process. She will need to rest until the pain settles, and should make a full recovery over the following days to weeks. A patient with a high fever (>38°C) or significant underlying medical problems may need to be admitted for monitoring, as he/she may be at risk of developing serious complications.

This woman should take a 7-day course of a regular non-steroidal anti-inflammatory drug (NSAID) such as ibuprofen. This will act to reduce inflammation and settle her chest pain. Patients who do not respond to a NSAID may need a course of corticosteroid.

Pericarditis can develop in the weeks following a myocardial infarction (Dressler's syndrome). As with other cases of pericarditis, this is usually self-limiting, and administration of a NSAID provides sufficient treatment. The presentation can be mistaken for a pulmonary embolism (sharp chest pain following a recent hospital admission) and so should always be considered following a recent myocardial infarction.

 KEY POINTS

- Pericarditis can present acutely or chronically. Pain is usually pleuritic and positional with characteristic ECG changes showing widespread saddle-shaped ST elevation.
- Most cases of acute pericarditis are viral and self-limiting.

CASE 41: FEVER IN A RETURNED TRAVELLER

History

A 28-year-old wildlife photographer returned to the UK two weeks ago after a short visit to Zambia. She has presented to her GP with a one-week history of relapsing and remitting fever, accompanied by a generalized headache and malaise which are becoming more severe and associated with excessive daytime somnolence. She is otherwise fit and well and has no drug history. She took a full course of malaria prophylaxis throughout and after her travels.

Examination

There are multiple excoriation marks all over her body. There are indurated tender ulcers with surrounding cellulitis in the left leg with associated left inguinal lymphadenopathy. The rest of the examination is unremarkable. Observations: temperature 37.6°C, heart rate 98/min, blood pressure 108/60 mmHg, SaO_2 100 per cent on room air.

INVESTIGATIONS		
		Normal range
White cells	24.0	$4–11 \times 10^9$/L
Haemoglobin	10.0	13–18 g/dL
Platelets	90	$150–400 \times 10^9$/L
Sodium	135	135–145 mmol/L
Potassium	3.6	3.5–5.0 mmol/L
Urea	5.0	3.0–7.0 mmol/L
Creatinine	60	60–110 µmol/L
C-reactive protein	140	<5 mg/L
Blood film × 3:	No malarial parasite present	
Cerebrospinal fluid examination:		
All normal except for CSF microscopy, which showed the presence of morula or Mott cells		

Questions

• What is the diagnosis?
• How should this condition be treated?

ANSWER 41

Assessment of fever in a returned traveller should include a detailed travel history. Areas visited, activities, dates of onset of illness, use of prophylaxis or precautions, insect bites or injuries, and source of food or water consumed are important details to note. In this scenario the area of travel, clinical picture and tests are all supportive of human African trypanosomiasis ('sleeping sickness').

There are two subtypes: *Trypanosoma brucei gambiense* and *Trypanosoma brucei rhodesiense*. The former is more common in residents of endemic areas and is extremely rare in visitors; the opposite is true for the latter subtype. Unlike *gambiense*, where clinical progression is in stages over 1–2 years, *rhodesiense* leads to rapid progression to death over 1–3 months without clear stages of the disease.

The natural history of human African trypanosomiasis can be divided into two stages: the haemolymphatic and the meningoencephalitic. After inoculation, trypanosome protozoa proliferate and induce a local lymphocytic inflammation. The trypanosomes spread to reticuloendothelial organs, leading to their enlargement, and clinically the haemolymphatic stage symptoms manifest as fever, flu-like symptoms, generalized lymphadenopathy and hepatosplenomegaly. Fevers which last for seven days may come and go; this is due to continual variation of the trypanosome glycoprotein leading to a variable human-host immune response. A transient macular rash may also develop. In *rhodesiense* infection it is more common to develop a painful chancre at the site of inoculation, so fluid from these chancres could be used to look for trypanosomes. The later encephalitic stage occurs due to central nervous system invasion, which leads to psychiatric disturbances, confusion, reversal of the normal sleep/wake cycle with excessive somnolence, motor disturbances (tremor and fasciculation, pyramidal tone and weakness, cerebellar signs), sensory deficits (deep hyperaesthesia, cranial nerve lesions, pruritis) and seizures.

Definitive antiprotozoa treatment depends on the subtype of African trypanosomes. *Gambiense* is treated with pentamidine or eflornithine, depending on the stage of illness. *Rhodesiense* is treated with suramin with or without melarsoprol and steroids, again depending on the stage of illness.

 KEY POINT

- A good, comprehensive travel history is essential in the assessment of fever in a returned traveller.

CASE 42: RED EYES AND SIGHT IMPAIRMENT

History

A 30-year-old man of Japanese descent has presented to the emergency department with a two-day history of bilateral red eyes with visual impairment. Over the past year he has had recurrent fever, weight loss, right knee pain, recurrent oral ulcers and genital ulcers over the scrotum, but earlier investigations did not yield a uniform diagnosis. He has no sexual history. He has been treated with warfarin on three occasions due to deep vein thrombosis.

Examination

There is a watery discharge from his eyes, with evidence of ciliary and conjunctival injection. The pupils are small and irregular in shape and size with evidence of synechiae. The pupils react to light sluggishly. Ophthalmoscopy is not possible owing to discomfort in bright light. He has a visual acuity of 6/9 bilaterally. There is no evidence of lymphadenopathy, but there are multiple aphthous ulcers in the oral cavity. There is a tender, nodular rash over the shins bilaterally, and his right knee joint has minimal effusion and limited movements. His cardiorespiratory, abdominal and neurological examinations are unremarkable.

INVESTIGATIONS		
		Normal range
White cells	14.0	4–11×10^9/L
Haemoglobin	10.0	13–18 g/dL
Platelets	300	150–400×10^9/L
Sodium	136	135–145 mmol/L
Potassium	3.5	3.5–5.0 mmol/L
Urea	3.7	3.0–7.0 mmol/L
Creatinine	85	60–110 µmol/L
C-reactive protein	120	<5 mg/L
Rheumatoid factor	Negative	
Antinuclear antibodies	Negative	

Questions

- How would you manage this man's red eyes?
- What is the unifying diagnosis of this man's condition?

ANSWER 42

As a rule of thumb, 'serious red eye conditions' present with redness predominately situated where blood vessels emerge from the depth of the eye; this is called ciliary injection. This man's eye examination findings are suggestive of anterior uveitis. The major concern here is the potential threat to sight. Topical steroids and mydriatics should be given for anterior uveitis, and the condition should be monitored closely as recurrent uveitis can lead to permanent blindness.

Recognizing the cause of anterior uveitis is important as a number of conditions are associated with it:

- seronegative arthropathies such as ankylosing spondylitis;
- Behçet's disease;
- inflammatory bowel disease;
- sarcoidosis;
- infection – toxoplasmosis, toxocariasis, herpes simplex, varicella zoster virus.

The collection of features including orogenital ulcers, monoarthritis, anterior uveitis, erythema nodosum and history of multiple venous thromboembolism is highly suggestive of Behçet's disease. Other features of this condition include central nervous system involvement, gastrointestinal tract ulcerations, glomerulonephritis and amyloidosis. The multi-system nature of this illness is reflected by the underlying pathology as a systemic vasculitis. The pethargy reaction – a skin reaction occurring 1–2 days after a needle puncture – is an important clinical diagnostic feature of Behçet's disease.

On top of the local treatment of the anterior uveitis, thalidomide and colchicine are a recognized treatment for orogenital ulceration. Venous thromboembolism should be managed by warfarin accordingly.

 KEY POINTS

- It is important to establish the underlying cause of acute uveitis.
- Acute uveitis is a sight-threatening condition that should be recognized and treated promptly.
- Behçet's syndrome is a systemic vasculitis that is difficult to diagnose and treat.

CASE 43: RASH AND FLU-LIKE SYMPTOMS

History
A 42-year-old man has presented to his GP with a one-week history of flu-like symptoms including general malaise, fever, headache, muscle aches and joint pains. He notes that his joint pains have moved from one joint to another over the past week. He also complains of multiple rashes on his lower limbs which started as papules and then evolved daily into large erythematous lesions with areas of paleness in the middle of these lesions. He has no medical history and there has been no recent travel history abroad. He works as a gamekeeper on Exmoor.

Examination
There is a small area of cellulitis over the left calf. On the right lower leg there are multiple annular target-like erythematous rashes that are 8 cm in diameter. On the left knee there is a large, tender erythematous swelling but no other joints are affected. The rest of the clinical examination is unremarkable. Observations: temperature 37.9°C, heart rate 100/min, blood pressure 120/80 mmHg, SaO_2 100 per cent on room air.

INVESTIGATIONS		
		Normal range
White cells	22.0	$4-11 \times 10^9$/L
Haemoglobin	15.0	13–18 g/dL
Platelets	178	$150-400 \times 10^9$/L
Sodium	136	135–145 mmol/L
Potassium	4.2	3.5–5.0 mmol/L
Urea	7.6	3.0–7.0 mmol/L
Creatinine	89	60–110 µmol/L
INR	1.0	0.9–1.1
Left knee joint aspirate:		
Appearance	Straw-coloured with translucent clarity	
Cell count	Presence of leucocytes (2000 cells/mm³)	
ECG:		
Sinus tachycardia rate 102/min		

Questions
- What is the likely diagnosis?
- What is the appropriate management?

The description is consistent with Lyme borreliosis, which is the most common human tick-borne zoonosis in the northern hemisphere. *Borrelia burgdorferi* is the most common type of spirochaete leading to Lyme disease in the UK. The transmitting vector is an Ixodid tick which normally feeds on large mammals and birds. Humans may be incidental hosts and infection typically occurs at the nymphal stage of its life cycle.

Primary prevention through appropriate clothing and the use of skin insect repellents containing *N,N*-diethyl-meta-toluamide (DEET) may reduce the risk of Lyme disease. Regular body checking for tick bites is also important. Not all tick bites are infective and antibiotic prophylaxis is not routinely recommended. Tick bite sufferers are normally advised to remove ticks with toothed tweezers and monitor for signs of erythema migrans (see below). Serological testing for asymptomatic individuals is also not recommended. The normal incubation period of Lyme is 1–2 weeks and not all patients infected with *Borrelia* are symptomatic. In suspected cases of Lyme disease it is usual to treat with antibiotics empirically; the recommended regimen in the UK is either amoxicillin or doxycycline. Serological testing is not always needed if presentation is typical. The timing of serological testing is important as most patients will be seropositive only 2–4 weeks after onset of symptoms, and even then the testing is not 100 per cent sensitive.

The presentation of Lyme disease varies greatly. Three-quarters of cases develop erythema migrans, with target-like erythematous lesions. These lesions may become chronic and develop into cellulitis-like lesions. Rarely, acrodermatitis chronica atrophicans – with chronic blue lesions – occurs and it typically affects the extensor surfaces of limbs accompanied by peripheral neuropathy. Another rare skin manifestation, which typically occurs in cases outside Europe, is borrelial lymphocytoma – with plaque-like lesions mimicking cutaneous lymphoma.

Other manifestations occur in the nervous system (bilateral cranial nerve 7 palsies, subacute lymphocytic meningitis/encephalitis, subacute demyelinating and axonal sensory/motor neuropathy causing severe radicular nerve root pain), cardiovascular system (myocarditis, second/third degree heart block) and arthropathies, which typically affect large joints causing large swelling but surprisingly little accompanying pain. If left untreated this arthropathy may become chronic.

 KEY POINTS

- Lyme borreliosis can potentially have multi-system manifestations.
- It is not always necessary to have a positive Lyme serology prior to initiation of treatment.

CASE 44: SUBSTANCE ABUSE AND AGITATION

History

A 20-year-old woman has been brought to the emergency department by her friends from the local nightclub. She is agitated, confused and verbally aggressive. The friends report a fitting episode lasting 30 seconds en route to the hospital. They also say that she has taken 'some pills'. She refuses to cooperate with staff and says she wants to dance.

Examination

She will not agree to a full examination, but cooperates enough for observations to be obtained: temperature 38°C, heart rate 130/min (regular), blood pressure 170/130 mmHg, SaO_2 99 per cent on room air. She is noted to have excessive diaphoresis and has grossly dilated pupils (size 5). She is very talkative and paces up and down the department.

Questions
- What are the differential diagnoses of this woman's presentation?
- What is the appropriate management?

The limited history suggests this woman may be intoxicated due to substance abuse. For various reasons it is often difficult to tell what substance a person has taken. Clues may be found in clinical examination and behavioural observation. In this scenario she appears agitated with dilated pupils. Her observations reveal hyperthermia, tachycardia and hypertension; these are signs of sympathomimetic or anticholinergic drug actions. Her hyperthermia is more in keeping with sympathomimetic poisoning (e.g. amphetamines or MDMA, also known as Ecstasy).

There are common steps in the management of acute intoxication and poisoning. As with most medical emergencies, the airway, breathing and circulation (ABC) should be assessed and managed appropriately in the first instance. Neurological examinations should be carried out to look for lateralizing and/or cerebellar signs. It is also important to examine for abnormal ocular movements and papillary changes as it helps to give clues to the common drugs/toxins involved. Blood glucose should be checked especially when a patient presents with a history of seizure activity. Naloxone should be given as intravenous bolus to diagnose opioid poisoning if this is suspected. Essential investigations of suspected poisoning include electrocardiogram, blood test for renal function, creatine kinase, liver function tests, calcium, bicarbonate and chloride levels. In practice some doctors would also consider measuring paracetamol and salicylate levels in any poisoning cases to screen for co-ingestion of drugs, especially in patients suspected to have attempted self-harm or suicide.

Often a 'drug screen' is requested but this is rarely necessary. A typical drug screen is expensive and difficult to interpret. The results may take 1–2 weeks to become available and it is not possible to screen for all possible toxins. Therefore it does not alter immediate patient management in most instances. A drug screen is sometimes used for medico-legal purposes.

Neuroimaging, such as CT of brain, is only necessary when patients are suspected to have a structural brain lesion or significant head injury. A provoked seizure from poisoning or substance abuse does not necessitate neuroimaging in most circumstances.

MDMA and amphetamines have a variable duration of clinical effects: the larger the dose ingested, the longer the clinical effects last. Tolerance is common and chronic abusers may take a much larger dose.

Important side-effects of these drugs are cardiac arrhythmia (supraventricular or ventricular), hyponatraemia (secondary to excess water consumption and excess secretion of antidiuretic hormone), cerebral haemorrhage (secondary to severe hypertension), seizure and a hyperthermic syndrome similar to serotonin syndrome which would lead to acute kidney injury, disseminated intravascular coagulation, rhabdomyolysis and hepatocellular necrosis.

In most instances MDMA or amphetamine toxicity is managed supportively. Volume status should be assessed; if dehydrated, intravenous fluid should be given. Cold intravenous fluid is also used to lower temperature in hyperthermic patients. Conversely, hyponatraemia should be managed by fluid restriction. Diazepam is used to manage agitation and hypertension.

KEY POINTS

- The recognition of different syndromes associated with common drug toxicity is essential to work out the underlying drug toxicity.
- A 'drug screen' is not needed in most cases of poisoning
- Beware of mixed poisoning and staggered overdose: always have a high index of suspicion.
- In most cases the treatment of poisonings requires supportive therapy only as specific antidotes are often not available. Liaise with the regional poisoning information centre as appropriate. Useful clinical advice is available on the internet at TOXBASE: www.toxbase.org/ .

History

A 25-year-old man has presented to his GP with a one-month history of a generalized rash and pruritis. This rash started on the trunk and has spread to all four limbs, neck and scalp. It is associated with malaise, recurrent fevers and sweatiness. There are no mucosal ulcers or eye disorders. He does not recall any recent sore throat or flu-like illness. There is no drug or travel history and he has no history of skin disorders. He works as a teacher and was fit and well prior to his present condition. However, he does have a one-year history of back pain in the lumbar area and left knee pain, and as a result he has been unable to play football regularly.

Examination

This man feels extremely warm to the touch. There is a symmetrical, generalized body rash covering most of the body area with coarse scaling. There is no lymphadenopathy and no mouth ulcers, but his tongue is dry. His jugular venous pressure (JVP) is not seen even when lying flat, and his pulse is hyperdynamic but regular. The rest of the cardiovascular, respiratory, abdominal and neurological examinations are unremarkable. Observations: temperature 37.7°C, heart rate 130/min, blood pressure 110/70 mmHg, respiratory rate 24/min, SaO_2 100 per cent on room air.

INVESTIGATIONS		
		Normal range
White cells	15.0	$4–11 \times 10^9$/L
Haemoglobin	11.4	13–18 g/dL
Platelets	180	$150–400 \times 10^9$/L
Sodium	133	135–145 mmol/L
Potassium	3.4	3.5–5.0 mmol/L
Urea	12	3.0–7.0 mmol/L
Creatinine	140	60–110 µmol/L
C-reactive protein	88	<5 mg/L

Questions
- What is the most likely diagnosis?
- What would be the appropriate management?

ANSWER 45

This young man has presented with a rash, low-grade fever and raised inflammatory markers. The generalized, scaly rash is typical for erythroderma. Other possible diagnoses could include a viral exanthem or a drug reaction (although there is no history of a new drug being introduced). Erythroderma is a clinical syndrome describing an erythematous rash involving more than 90 per cent of the skin. This is a potentially life-threatening syndrome as the extent of the rash can lead to skin failure: the skin is unable to maintain core temperature, retain fluid and to defend against infections.

A range of skin diseases can potentially lead to erythroderma, the most common being psoriasis, eczema and drug reactions, and rarely severe skin infections and T-cell lymphoma. Management includes general supportive care of skin failure (similar to that for a burns victim) as well as diagnosis and treatment of the underlying cause.

The diagnosis of the underlying cause of erythroderma should include a detailed history of the rash. A rapid onset with no preceding history may suggest an acute infection, allergy to environmental factors or drugs. Usually erythrodermic patients have had a skin disease such as psoriasis or atopic eczema. A detailed drug and travel history should be recorded. Skin biopsies are often carried out when the diagnosis is unclear clinically. Cutaneous T-cell lymphoma is difficult to diagnose and multiple skin biopsies are often done in order to firmly establish the diagnosis. The treatment of underlying severe psoriasis may involve an immunosuppressive agent such as methotrexate.

In this case the psoriasiform nature of the rash and history of preceding arthropathy point towards psoriasis as the underlying cause of his erythroderma.

General supportive care includes the following:

- Take steps to maintain the core temperature to prevent hypothermia.
- Stop all unnecessary medications.
- Give dietary supplements to support nutrition, as erythrodermic patients are in high catabolic state.
- Minimize the extent of intravenous access as much as possible.
- Give thromboprophylaxis unless clearly contraindicated.
- Assess fluid status by clinical examination and daily weighing to maintain good hydration, and manage renal failure accordingly.
- Monitor closely for clinical deterioration as secondary sepsis is very common. Culture and manage with antibiotics.
- Prevent stress ulcers by proton pump inhibitors.
- Avoid blood glucose >10 mmol/L and manage with intravenous insulin accordingly.
- Give frequent attention to skin care. Apply emollients such as soft paraffin. Avoid adhesive tapes in affected skin areas. Frequently turn sedated/immobilized patients.
- Swab all affected areas frequently to look for bacterial superinfection and treat sepsis early and aggressively.
- Consider ophthalmic referral if the underlying cause has ophthalmic complications (e.g. toxic epidermal necrolysis).
- Pain and itching are often difficult to manage. Generous use of opioids and sedating antihistamines may be necessary.

KEY POINTS

- Erythroderma is a clinical syndrome with a rash covering more than 90 per cent of the body.
- There is often a history of a previous skin disease, such as psoriasis or eczema.

CASE 46: PRURITIC RASH AND ALOPECIA

History
A 68-year-old man has presented to his GP with a red scaly rash over his body. For about five years he has had multiple, intensely itchy, red scaly patches over his trunk. Despite skin biopsies on several occasions, the histological diagnosis of his condition remains inconclusive. A trial of a potent topical steroid in the past did not affect the patches. Over the past two weeks most areas of his body have become erythematous.

Examination
Cardiovascular and respiratory examinations are unremarkable. Abdominal examination reveals hepatosplenomegaly, and large lymph nodes are present in the axillary and cervical regions. Mucous membranes are normal. The entire surface area of the skin is diffusely erythematous. Palms and soles are thickened and there is total alopecia. Observations: temperature 37.2°C, heart rate 110/min, blood pressure 90/60 mmHg, SaO_2 96 per cent on room air.

INVESTIGATIONS		
		Normal range
White cells	15.0	$4–11 \times 10^9$/L
Haemoglobin	9.4	13–18 g/dL
Platelets	100	$150–400 \times 10^9$/L
Sodium	133	135–145 mmol/L
Potassium	3.4	3.5–5.0 mmol/L
Urea	18	3.0–7.0 mmol/L
Creatinine	200	60–110 µmol/L
C-reactive protein	88	<5 mg/L

Questions
- What is the unifying diagnosis?
- What should be the immediate management?

ANSWER 46

The history suggests that this man's rash has been going on for several years. The examination findings of hepatosplenomegaly and lymphadenopathy suggest an underlying disease process infiltrating lymphoid organs. The findings are highly suggestive of chronic cutaneous T-cell lymphoma, also known as mycosis fungoides or Sézary syndrome (when there is haematogenous dissemination of clonal T-cells). The T-cells involved are the CLA+ cells, which home to skin tissues and are usually CD4+ T-cells. This is a rare disorder and can be complicated by erythroderma at any stage of the illness.

Definitive diagnosis can be difficult and multiple biopsies may remain inconclusive for many years. Staging of this disease depends on the tumour load in skin, blood, lymph node and visceral organs: the management plan is dependent on the staging results. The general management of an acutely unwell erythrodermic patient is mentioned elsewhere in this book (see case 45).

Owing to the wide variability in the presentation and natural history of this illness, treatment algorithms are not standardized. Possible treatment options are topical steroids, phototherapy, chemotherapy, radiotherapy, retinoids, photopheresis, immunobiological therapies and bone marrow transplant in selected cases.

Cutaneous T-cell lymphoma is an indolent illness that is not curable and can last for many years. However, patients with Sézary syndrome have a poorer prognosis with a median survival of 1–3 years.

 KEY POINTS

- Mycosis fungoides is a cutanous T-cell lymphoma, presenting with infiltration of lymphoid organs and skin changes.
- The diagnosis can be difficult to make and the disease can be very extensive by the time the diagnosis is reached.

History

A 24-year-old woman has presented to the emergency department with a reduction in visual acuity of her right eye, developing over the past few days. This is associated with pain on right eye movement, and she describes a reduction in colour vision in the same eye. She denies any headache or other neurological symptoms.

Examination

This young woman's right and left eye visual acuities are 6/24 and 6/6 respectively. Examination of the visual fields reveals a central scotoma. There is a relative afferent pupillary defect on the right eye. Fundoscopy reveals a normal optic disc. The rest of the cardiorespiratory, abdominal and neurological examinations are unremarkable.

Questions
- What is the diagnosis?
- How can this condition be managed?

ANSWER 47

Presentation of reduced visual acuity and colour vision is typical of any optic neuropathy (except for papilloedema: usually patients suffering from papilloedema do not complain of reduced visual acuity). In common with all optic neuropathies, there is a varying degree of relative afferent pupillary defect and central scotoma. It is also important to perform fundoscopy to exclude retinal pathologies (e.g. retinal detachment) which can present in a similar way. In this scenario the patient is likely to have experienced an episode of optic neuritis or retrobulbar neuritis.

When patients over the age of 50 years present with symptoms of optic neuropathy, it is essential to ask whether there has been any history of headache or polymyalgia symptoms (e.g. shoulder and/or pelvic girdle pain) and to measure the erythrocyte sedimentation rate (ESR) to exclude temporal arteritis. Although rare, severe sphenoidal sinusitis can also present with a sudden reduction in visual acuity and colour vision and pain on eye movement. If this is suspected, an urgent CT of the sinus cavities and an ENT opinion should be sought.

Optic neuritis typically affects young females and rarely presents over the age of 45 years. The classical presenting symptoms are of unilateral loss of visual acuity and pain on eye movement. It is usually self-limiting, with full function returning within three months. Fifty per cent of patients will develop a second episode of optic neuritis and this is highly suggestive of multiple sclerosis, which should be further investigated. It is therefore important that the presence of paraesthesia, dizziness, shooting neck pain or limb weakness and Uthoff's phenomenon (worsening of neurological symptoms in warm conditions, e.g. a hot bath) guide you towards the diagnosis of multiple sclerosis in patients who present with optic neuritis.

The treatment of optic neuritis with agents such as steroids remains controversial. It is best to refer to local policy and follow specialist advice.

 KEY POINTS

- Optic neuritis presents with pain, loss of vision and a reduction in colour vision (particularly the colour red).
- Optic neuritis is often a feature of multiple sclerosis, so a full history must be taken and a neurological examination should be performed.

History

A 26-year-old woman has presented to the emergency department with a two-day history of anorexia, malaise and fever. She is normally fit and well, but over the past 24 hours she has been experiencing a constant right iliac fossa pain radiating to her right flank, increasing in severity. This was preceded by urinary frequency and dysuria, but there has been no recent change in bowel habit.

Examination

This woman is not icteric and there is no lymphadenopathy. Her cardiorespiratory examination is unremarkable. On palpation of her abdomen, there is tenderness over the right side and the right flank. There is no rebound tenderness. Bowel sounds are normal. Rectal examination reveals an empty rectum. An erect chest X-ray is normal, but an abdominal X-ray shows a non-specific large bowel gas pattern. Observations: temperature 39°C, heart rate 110/min, blood pressure 100/60 mmHg, respiratory rate 24/min, SaO_2 100 per cent on room air.

INVESTIGATIONS		
		Normal range
White cells	18.0	$4–11 \times 10^9$/L
Haemoglobin	15.6	13–18 g/dL
Platelets	208	$150–400 \times 10^9$/L
Sodium	134	135–145 mmol/L
Potassium	3.5	3.5–5.0 mmol/L
Urea	4.0	3.0–7.0 mmol/L
Creatinine	86	60–110 μmol/L
C-reactive protein	120	<5 mg/L
Amylase	88	30–110 IU/L
Urine dipstick:		
– Protein	2+	
– Blood	2+	
– Nitrite	Positive	
– Leu	4+	
Urinary pregnancy test	Negative	

Questions

- What is the differential diagnosis?
- What other information would you gather to confirm the diagnosis?
- How would you manage this woman?

The differential diagnosis of a young woman presenting with right iliac fossa pain includes appendicitis, Crohn's disease, ovarian torsion, mesenteric adenitis, ectopic pregnancy, and renal and ureteric pathologies such as pyelonephritis and/or obstructing renal calculi.

The history-taking should include menstrual and sexual information. Per vaginal bleeding preceded by abdominal pain with positive pregnancy test should prompt urgent referral to a gynaecologist for the management of suspected ectopic pregnancy.

Ovarian torsion and appendicitis can potentially present similarly, but the presence of urinary symptoms and positive urine dipstick is highly suggestive of pyelonephritis.

In this case, the woman had symptoms of fever, dysuria and abdominal pain. Her urine results are consistent with a urinary tract infection and she can be diagnosed with pyelonephritis. This is a urinary tract infection that has ascended up to the renal pelvis. Diagnosis is usually made on the basis of symptoms of rigors, dysuria, iliac fossa or loin tenderness and vomiting, as well as signs of systemic infection (fever, tachycardia and hypotension). The urine dip is usually positive for nitrites (produced by certain bacteria) and leucocytes. Pyelonephritis is commonly caused by Gram-negative organisms and empirical antibiotics should be given according to the local policy. Blood and urine cultures should be taken as soon as possible, but this should not delay the administration of antibiotics. Intravenous fluid should be considered in hypovolaemic and/or septic patients. Urinary output should be monitored. Ultrasound of the renal tract should be considered to look for evidence of hydronephrosis, emphysematous pyelitis or abscesses – all of which would need urgent urology consultation.

Most women will experience a urinary tract infection (UTI) at some time in their life, so education towards UTI prevention is important (e.g. wipe from front to back after a bowel movement or after urinating, and try to empty the bladder before and after sexual intercourse).

 KEY POINTS

- Many pathologies can present with right iliac fossa pain. It is important to learn how to differentiate one from another.
- In female patients of child-bearing age, a pregnancy test should be performed to ensure an ectopic pregnancy is not missed.

History

A 62-year-old woman has presented to the emergency department with a one-week history of painful right shoulder. She suffers from aggressive rheumatoid arthritis with multiple joint involvement. She has previously complained of right shoulder joint stiffness, but over the past week she has been unable to move her shoulder owing to severe pain. This is associated with worsening general malaise. Her medical history includes stage 3 chronic kidney disease. She takes methotrexate 10 mg once a week and ramipril 5 mg daily.

Examination

This woman is obese, but cardiorespiratory and abdominal examinations are unremarkable. Her right shoulder joint is tender on palpation, and no active or passive movements are possible because of pain. There is mild erythema over the right shoulder and it feels slightly warm to the touch. A shoulder X-ray reveals osteopenic bones but no joint abnormality is detected. Observations: temperature 37.9°C, heart rate 92/min, blood pressure 100/65 mmHg, SaO_2 93 per cent on room air.

INVESTIGATIONS		
		Normal range
White cells	8.0	$4-11 \times 10^9$/L
Haemoglobin	9.0	13–18 g/dL
Platelets	155	$150-400 \times 10^9$/L
Sodium	135	135–145 mmol/L
Potassium	3.7	3.5–5.0 mmol/L
Urea	9	3.0–7.0 mmol/L
Creatinine	120	60–110 µmol/L
C-reactive protein	46	<5 mg/L

Questions
- What are the main differential diagnoses in this case?
- What would be your immediate management plan?

The main differential diagnoses of this woman's presentation are septic arthritis, pathological fracture, crystal arthropathies or acute flare of rheumatoid arthritis. Septic arthritis should be suspected in any patient with rheumatoid arthritis with sudden onset or worsening of joint symptoms. Clinical signs of septic arthritis may be atypical or may not reflect the severity due to concomitant immunosuppressive therapy – in this case with methotrexate. There is an increased risk of pathological or low-impact fractures in rheumatoid arthritis owing to the underlying inflammatory process, inactivity, and steroid and methotrexate use.

It is prudent to rule out septic arthritis in the first instance. Obtain blood tests to look for raised inflammatory markers and to look for other target damage such as chronic kidney disease which may be relevant in a multi-system disorder associated with frequent use of immunosuppressives.

Interpretation of C-reactive protein (CRP) and erythrocyte sedimentation rate (ESR) may be difficult, particularly the ESR. Chronic anaemia is common in patients with rheumatoid arthritis, and ESR is raised in anaemia. Both CRP and ESR could be raised due to underlying inflammation, or they could be mildly raised only due to immunosuppressive therapy.

There is some evidence to support the use of procalcitonin in patients with autoimmune disorders to help identify bacterial sepsis. Blood culture should be obtained if pyrexial. Joint aspiration should be carried out as soon as possible but should not delay the administration of empirical antibiotics. Joint aspirate should be sent for microscopy for bacteria and culture and for crystal identification. If a prosthetic joint is involved then aspiration should be carried out in an operating theatre by an orthopaedic surgeon.

Once the diagnosis of septic arthritis is confirmed, a joint washout should be considered. In this scenario methotrexate should be withdrawn temporarily. Pain management is important, so paracetamol and opioids should be considered as appropriate.

 KEY POINTS

- Patients with known rheumatoid arthritis presenting with acute joint pain should be investigated for septic arthritis.
- If the diagnosis of septic arthritis is confirmed, a joint washout should be considered.
- Pain management is important, so paracetamol and opioids should be considered as appropriate.

CASE 50: FACIAL RASH

History

A 34-year-old woman has presented to her GP with a one-day history of high fever, lethargy and a rapidly spreading rash over the malar bones and nasal bridges. She has a five-year history of systemic lupus erythematosus (SLE) that had initially presented with inflammation and pain of the small joints of the hands, but this is now well-controlled by hydroxychloroquine. She has been monitored by a rheumatologist over the past five years and, apart from a mild anaemia, she has had no other systemic features of SLE. She does not have a history of recent foreign travel.

Examination

This woman is warm to the touch, her pulse is bounding and she looks unwell. Over the nasal bridge and malar bones there is a well-demarcated erythematous plaque that is tender. There are no oral lesions but there are multiple small cervical lymph nodes. The rest of the examination is unremarkable. Observations: temperature 38.7°C, heart rate 110/min, blood pressure 100/60 mmHg, respiratory rate 24/min, SaO_2 96 per cent on room air.

INVESTIGATIONS		
		Normal range
White cells	15.0	$4–11 \times 10^9$/L
Haemoglobin	10.0	13–18 g/dL
Platelets	100	$150–400 \times 10^9$/L
Sodium	137	135–145 mmol/L
Potassium	4.1	3.5–5.0 mmol/L
Urea	10	3.0–7.0 mmol/L
Creatinine	140	60–110 µmol/L
C-reactive protein	120	<5 mg/L
Erythrocyte sedimentation rate	100 mm/h	Male: age/2
		Female: (age+10)/2

Question

- How would you manage this woman?

ANSWER 50

Systemic lupus erythematosus is a complex multi-system disorder that carries excess mortality. The majority of SLE patients have a natural history of episodic exacerbations or flares. Sometimes remissions may be prolonged and the pattern of exacerbations is usually established within 5–10 years of disease onset. If aggressive SLE flares occur frequently and early in the disease course, then mortality risk is high. Most patients tend to die of premature cardiovascular disease (stroke, ischaemic heart disease), renal disease or sepsis.

When reviewing a patient with a history of SLE, the main focus is to decide whether the presentation is due to a flare or to a complication of SLE such as infection or an unrelated condition. In this scenario it is important to decide whether the rash is a photosensitive 'butterfly' rash that occurs in one-third of SLE patients, or is due to erysipelas/facial cellulitis. Important information to elicit is whether this woman has ever had a similar rash, or a change in cosmetic product, facial trauma or increased sun exposure.

The history of a rapidly spreading facial demarcated rash in a systemically unwell patient with high C-reactive protein (CRP) should raise suspicion of facial erysipelas. Classically, CRP is relatively normal and the erythrocyte sedimentation rate (ESR) is markedly raised in acute SLE flares, so a markedly raised CRP in this case suggests an active infection. Procalcitonin may have a role in the management of this condition, both to aid diagnosis of bacterial infection and to aid decisions regarding antibiotic therapy.

A rheumatology consultation should be sought. In some instances, complement level and anti-double stranded DNA antibody titre may be useful as they correlate with SLE disease activity. In this scenario, blood cultures should be taken and antibiotics and fluid resuscitation should be instigated without any delay. Rapid improvement should be expected, otherwise it is important to look out for intracranial complications such as cavernous sinus thrombosis and orbital cellulitis – known important complications of facial cellulitis.

 KEY POINTS

- An acute SLE flare should be differentiated from other complications such as sepsis in an acutely unwell patient.
- If aggressive SLE flares occur frequently and early in the disease course, then mortality risk is high.

CASE 51: A WOMAN 'OFF HER LEGS'

History

An 82-year-old woman has been referred by her GP for confusion and being 'off her legs'. She appears vacant and is unable to say why and how she came to the hospital. The referral letter states that she lives alone and has no immediate family. She was previously independent and walked with the aid of two sticks. Her medical history includes hypertension and osteoporosis. She is taking amlodipine 10 mg once daily and risedronate 35 mg once per week.

Examination

This elderly woman appears thin but healthy and well hydrated. There is a recent moderate sized cut above her left eye and there are several cuts and bruising on her arms and shins. She is unable to perform the 'get up and go' test as she is unable to stand up. She is orientated in person only and is easily distracted by the surroundings, making physical examination very difficult. Her cardiovascular, respiratory and abdominal examinations are unremarkable. There is no evidence of neck stiffness or photophobia. Her pupils are equal and dilated and there are no abnormalities on examination of her cranial nerves. In her peripheral nervous system there is normal tone but globally depressed power (4/5). Reflexes are difficult to elicit and she is unable to carry out clinical tests for coordination. Plantars are both withdrawn. Fundoscopy is within normal limits. A chest X-ray shows no abnormal features. Observations: temperature 36.8°C, heart rate 80/min, blood pressure 138/65 mmHg, SaO_2 97 per cent on room air.

INVESTIGATIONS		
		Normal range
White cells	8.0	$4–11 \times 10^9$/L
Haemoglobin	12.8	13–18 g/dL
Platelets	250	$150–400 \times 10^9$/L
Sodium	125	135–145 mmol/L
Potassium	3.7	3.5–5.0 mmol/L
Urea	14.5	3.0–7.0 mmol/L
Creatinine	76	60–110 µmol/L
C-reactive protein	<5	<5 mg/L
Corrected calcium	2.2	2.2–2.6 mmol/L
Urine sodium	21 mmol/L	
Urine dipstick	1+ protein	

Questions

- How would you interpret the low serum sodium?
- What are the possible differential diagnoses for this woman's presentation?

ANSWER 51

The low serum sodium interpreted with continued urinary sodium excretion is highly suggestive of the syndrome of inappropriate antidiuretic hormone secretion (SIADH). To make the diagnosis it is necessary to ensure this patient is clinically euvolaemic without any other precipitants of hyponatraemia, such as diarrhoea and vomiting or diuretic use. The causes of SIADH are wide and can be classified into:

- increased hypothalamic ADH production (cerebral trauma, infection, space-occupying lesion);
- drugs – diuretics (which cause sodium depletion), chlorpropamide, carbamazepine, non-steroidal anti-inflammatories, tricyclic antidepressants, selective serotonin-reuptake inhibitors (SSRIs), typical antipsychotics, monoamine oxidase inhibitors, chemotherapeutic agents;
- pulmonary diseases (carcinoma, pneumonia);
- exogenous administration of ADH;
- idiopathic.

This woman presented with delirium which is one of the geriatric giants. Her 'get up and go' test may be difficult to interpret owing to her confusional state, but it would suggest a limited mobility and underlying risk of falling. Her physical signs of recent head trauma and bruising support a history of recent fall(s). Information from history, examination and investigation results did not show any common precipitating causes of delirium, such as infection, intoxications or metabolic derangements. Intracranial pathologies such as post-ictal state or space-occupying lesion may possibly explain her current presentation. Her clinical neurological signs are difficult to interpret: global weakness could be related to hyponatraemia, and confusion often makes eliciting neurological signs difficult.

As part of the work-up for her delirium it may be useful to obtain neuroimaging such as a CT brain to look for evidence of a space-occupying lesion, such as sub-dural haematoma or gliomas. If this test is negative it may be worthwhile considering other tests such as EEG or lumbar puncture to exclude other intracranial causes of delirium. In this case a CT scan of the brain showed a right subdural haematoma (Fig. 51.1).

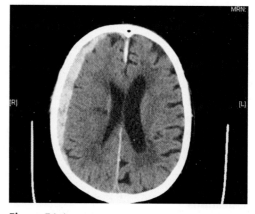

Figure 51.1

Collateral history is paramount to differentiate whether a presenting complaint of cognitive impairment is due to acute or chronic confusional state.

 KEY POINTS

- The diagnosis of syndrome of inappropriate antidiuretic hormone secretion should be made only after the patient's fluid status has been assessed.
- A subdural haematoma can present insidiously in the elderly as delirium.

CASE 52: ACUTE CONFUSION

History

A 65-year-old woman was found wandering the streets in a confused and agitated state, so passers-by called for an ambulance. The person was unable to give a thorough history. Her neighbours informed the paramedics that she was usually fit and well, although her medical history was significant for bipolar affective disorder, for which she takes lithium. Her other regular medications are ramipril and bendroflumethiazide for hypertension. She lives alone and attends a drop-in community mental health centre in addition to regular visits by a community psychiatric nurse and a friend. She denies smoking or alcohol intake.

Examination

No injuries are visible. Her mucous membranes appear dry. Cardiovascular, respiratory and abdominal examinations are unremarkable. There is a marked coarse tremor in all four limbs, symmetrically increased tone in the lower limbs, and an extrapyramidal gait. Her lithium level is 3 mmol/L. An ECG is shown in Fig. 52.1. Observations: temperature 37.4°C, heart rate 42/min, blood pressure 128/84 mmHg, respiratory rate 20/min, SaO_2 99 per cent on room air.

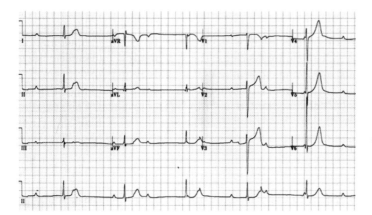

Figure 52.1

Questions

- What is the most likely diagnosis?
- What signs and symptoms should you be cautious of?
- What does the ECG show?
- How would you manage this patient acutely?

The patient is on lithium, so toxicity should always be suspected. Lithium toxicity occurs at levels greater than 1.4 mmol/L. Patients are particularly prone to developing lithium toxicity when they are dehydrated (e.g. secondary to diarrhoea or vomiting), or if they have renal impairment. Use of sodium-depleting drugs, such as thiazide diuretics and angiotensin-converting enzyme inhibitors, can also predispose a person to lithium toxicity.

Symptoms of lithium toxicity usually begin with gastrointestinal disturbances, such as nausea, vomiting and diarrhoea. This can then progress to neurological symptoms of ataxia and confusion. The person may have hyper-reflexia, hypertonia and nystagmus. People can experience seizures and eventually progress to coma. Cardiotoxicity is common.

This woman's ECG shows third-degree atrioventricular block, also known as complete heart block. The P waves show a regular P–P interval. The QRS complexes also demonstrate a regular R–R interval. The P–R interval is variable and there appears to be no relationship between the P waves and the QRS complexes. This is because the impulses generated by the sinoatrial node do not propagate down to the ventricles and the rhythms of the atria and the ventricles are completely dissociated. Because the sinoatrial node cannot conduct to the ventricles, an accessory pacemaker site further down the cardiac tissue will usually develop and activate the ventricles, leading to an escape rhythm.

Lithium overdose can lead to cardiotoxicity. First-degree heart block, where the duration of the P–R interval is increased, commonly develops. This can progress to complete heart block, as in this case. Patients with complete heart block are at high risk for hypotensive, bradycardic episodes and life-threatening arrhythmias. This woman should be placed on a cardiac monitor to observe her cardiac rhythm and may need a temporary pacing wire to be sited.

Your focus will be to prevent seizures and the development of renal failure or cardiotoxicity. Lithium is completely absorbed by the gastrointestinal tract and then renally excreted.

Owing to the complete heart block, the patient is at risk of further abnormal rhythms, including asystole.

Those with mild lithium toxicity (1.5–2.5 mmol/L) who appear clinically well and are asymptomatic should be monitored closely. Ensure that the patient is passing good volumes of urine. Increased oral intake of fluid and possibly intravenous fluids may be necessary.

People with lithium levels above 2.5 mmol/L will need to be admitted to hospital for inpatient management. The patient should be placed on a cardiac monitor and senior medical staff should be involved early.

If the overdose was taken within the last few hours, advice should be sought from a poisons centre as to whether methods such as gastric lavage or whole-bowel irrigation are recommended. Activated charcoal ingestion offers no benefit with lithium as the ions do not bind to the charcoal. Intravenous fluid therapy must be commenced early and haemodialysis should be considered to remove the lithium from the circulation. Drugs to alkalinize the urine may help to improve lithium excretion.

Lithium levels in the blood will need to be monitored frequently. If the patient is not improving, his/her care should be escalated to a high-dependency unit or intensive-care setting.

KEY POINTS

- Monitor lithium levels in patients using this drug. Lithium toxicity can be very dangerous, leading to multi-organ failure.
- When a person presents with lithium toxicity, involve senior doctors early.
- Perform blood tests to check renal function and ensure the patient stays on a cardiac monitor if he/she has ECG abnormalities or symptoms suggesting cardiac dysfunction.
- Dialysis may be required.

History

A 75-year-old man has been found on the ground by his neighbour and brought to the emergency department. The man appears unkept, confused and agitated. His only complaint is of numb feet and he appears unsteady. Once a week his neighbour checks on him but generally he likes to be left alone. The neighbour has noticed that the man's memory has been worsening lately. It is unclear what medications he might be taking, but the neighbour recalls he is a diabetic and takes 'a tablet' for this. He is not known to drink alcohol but does smoke. He is known to be a vegetarian.

Examination

This elderly man appears pale and is now unable to stand. There are several petechiae. He has glossitis and angular cheilitis. Cardiovascular, respiratory and abdominal examinations are unremarkable. Assessment of cognitive function shows a reduced abbreviated mental test score of 5/10. There is distal weakness affecting all limbs. Plantar responses are extensor. Knee and ankle jerks are absent. He is too confused to undergo testing of vibration sense and joint position sense. He refuses ophthalmoscopy. Observations: temperature 37.0°C, blood pressure 125/62 mmHg, heart rate 62/min, respiratory rate 20/min, SaO$_2$ 96 per cent on room air.

INVESTIGATIONS		
		Normal range
White cells	4.0	4–11 × 10⁹/L
Haemoglobin	6.5	13–18 g/dL
Mean cell volume	115	78–100 fL
Platelets	130	150–400 × 10⁹/L
Sodium	138	135–145 mmol/L
Potassium	3.8	3.5–5.0 mmol/L
Urea	4.0	3.0–7.0 mmol/L
Creatinine	48	60–110 µmol/L
C-reactive protein	300	<5 mg/L
Bilirubin	52	5–25 µmol/L
Alanine aminotransferase	24	8–55 IU/L
Alkaline phosphatase	150	42–98 IU/L
Albumin	32	35–50 g/L
Glucose	10.9	3.5–5.5 mmol/L
Intrinsic factor antibody	Positive	
Antiparietal cell antibody	Positive	

Questions:

- What do these findings suggest, and how would you confirm the diagnosis?
- How would you manage this patient?

ANSWER 53

This patient has a low haemoglobin and an elevated mean cell volume (MCV), making this a macrocytic anaemia. There are many causes of an elevated MCV, including haemolytic anaemia (large numbers of reticulocytes), as well as any cause of B_{12} or folate deficiency.

He has a distal weakness and absent knee and ankle reflexes, suggesting a peripheral motor neuropathy. It is unclear whether he has prominent sensory symptoms also, but he does complain of numb feet. The combination of a severe macrocytic anaemia and neurological signs suggests vitamin B_{12} deficiency.

Several differentials do exist in this case particularly as he is confused and unable to give a complete history. Alcoholic liver disease can present with macrocytic anaemia and nutritional deficiencies. Hypothyroidism can be excluded by a normal thyroid-stimulating hormone (TSH) level. He has a history of diabetes and his peripheral neuropathy may be caused by this; but it does not explain the worsening confusion and anaemia. Other causes of a macrocytic anaemia include folate deficiency, drugs (methotrexate, azathioprine) and myelodysplastic syndromes.

B_{12} deficiency is diagnosed by measuring the level of serum B_{12}. Less than 200 pg/mL is significant. Levels between 201 and 350 pg/mL require further testing. A peripheral blood film will show megalocytes (red blood cell precursors) with hypersegmented polymorphonuclear cells. The reticulocyte count will be low which suggests decreased production of red blood cells. Severe B_{12} deficiency can give rise to cognitive impairment or dementia, subacute combined degeneration of the spinal cord and optic atrophy. Other symptoms and signs are related to the degree of anaemia.

The acute management is to ensure haemodynamic stability and identify any signs to indicate that blood tranfusion is required (presence of heart failure, shortness of breath, chest pain). Patients who have severe anaemia are likely to need a blood transfusion but this has to be done cautiously due to the risk of precipitating heart failure. There are no signs of active bleeding and his blood pressure and heart rate are stable. There is no fever or raised inflammatory markers. Identifying the cause of his macrocytic anaemia is crucial to enable appropriate treatment. It is important to try to gain collateral history from the GP as past medical history and medications may help diagnose the cause.

Once a low vitamin B_{12} is established he should be given immediate intramuscular hydroxycobalamin as he has severe haematological and neurological features (peripheral neuropathy and pyramidal tract weakness with confusion). The usual dose is 1000 µg intramuscularly three times per week for two weeks, followed by once every three months.

Identifying the cause of vitamin B_{12} deficiency is the next step after urgently replacing it. In this case both intrinsic factor (IF) and antiparietal cell (APC) antibodies are positive. IF antibody is highly specific but only present in 50 per cent of cases. APC antibody is highly sensitive but not specific. Thus pernicious anaemia is the likely cause of vitamin B_{12} deficiency. Pernicious anaemia is an autoimmune condition where there is destruction of the gastric parietal cells that make IF. Other causes to know about are:

- reduced dietary intake (vegan diets, gastric/intestinal surgery);
- malabsorption from the GI tract (Crohn's, coeliac, bacterial overgrowth);
- proton pump inhibitors (reduce breakdown of vitamin B_{12} from food);
- metformin (decreases absorption of vitamin B_{12});
- atrophic gastritis.

CASE 54: POSTOPERATIVE HYPOTENSION

History

A 65-year-old man underwent an elective abdominal aortic aneurysm repair. He had a medical history of heart failure secondary to ischaemic heart disease, chronic renal impairment and type 2 diabetes mellitus.

Postoperative complications

Postoperatively this man developed acute abdominal pain and became hypotensive with a systolic blood pressure between 55 and 60 mmHg. He was given fluid resuscitation and required noradrenaline to keep his blood pressure elevated. His blood pressure remained low for about 30 minutes before it responded to fluids and vasopressors. He was oliguric. A haemoglobin from the blood gas machine was 5.5 g/dL. He was taken to surgery to repair a leak in the aortic graft and transfused 6 units of blood perioperatively. He remained oliguric for 24 hours until his renal function was repeated on day 3.

INVESTIGATIONS				
	Pre-op	Day 1 post-op	Day 3 post-op	Normal range
Na	138	131	129	135–145 mmol/L
K	4.8	5.8	6.5	3.5–5.0 mmol/L
Urea	15	28	32	3.0–7.0 mmol/L
Creatinine	140	280	335	60–110 µmol/L

Questions

- What is the cause of this man's acute renal impairment?
- What is the management of acute renal failure and hyperkalaemia?

ANSWER 54

The most likely cause of the renal impairment is renal failure secondary to hypovolaemia from an acute haemorrhage. The patient also has existing renal impairment, diabetes and coronary artery disease, all of which make him more at risk of renal hypoperfusion.

Acute renal failure (ARF; also known as acute kidney injury) is defined as an acute decline in glomerular filtration rate (GFR) from the baseline. The exact rise varies between guidelines. The RIFLE classification of ARF uses the level of rise in creatinine as a marker of the extent of renal damage. Urine output can be increased, decreased or absent. ARF is associated with increased mortality.

The main causes of ARF can be usefully categorized into pre-, intrinsic and post-renal. The main pre-renal cause is impaired blood flow to the kidneys from hypovolaemia, haemorrhage, dehydration or sepsis. Intrinsic renal causes include nephrotoxic drugs, interstitial nephritis or glomerular disease. Outflow obstructions from stones, enlarged prostate or masses are post-renal causes.

By day 3, this patient has developed hyperkalaemia and worsening renal function. Initial investigation should be directed at determining a diagnosis (in this case the most likely cause is hypovolaemia from an acute haemorrhage) and treating complications. Renal ultrasound is useful as it will determine whether there is an obstructive cause.

Immediately after the operation he did receive fluid resuscitation and vasopressor support, but his kidneys were not perfused adequately for at least 30 minutes. Urgent management was to stop the haemorrhage and transfuse with blood products. Now the focus should be on maintaining euvolaemia to ensure intravascular volume is adequate to perfuse the kidneys. In this case, optimizing cardiac output and volume status presents an additional challenge in view of his pre-existing renal impairment and heart failure. A crystalloid such as 0.9% saline is acceptable. The exact volume of replacement should be decided on parameters such as mean arterial pressure, cardiac index and other invasive monitoring available. The use of vasopressors and inotropes may be required to maintain renal perfusion pressures. Caution with intravascular volume replacement is necessary as he already has a history of heart failure and overfilling can impair cardiac function further. Invasive monitoring of central venous pressure, central venous saturations and cardiac index is therefore required in the setting of an intensive-care unit.

An ECG should be performed to identify any rhythm abnormalities associated with hyperkalaemia (Fig. 54.1). ECG signs of hyperkalaemia are tenting of the T waves, loss of P waves, widening of the QRS complex, VT or VF. In this case, the ECG showed absent P waves, a wide QRS complex and tall, tented T waves. Treatment is required if the potassium level is above 6.0 mmol/L with ECG changes. Initial treatments include administration of 10 mL of 10% calcium chloride or gluconate to stabilize the cardiac membrane. The effects are temporary and treatment can be repeated after 10 minutes. Intravenous insulin and dextrose should be administered to drive potassium intracellularly. This can lower potassium levels by about 0.5–1 mmol/L and last up to two hours. Therefore, it may often need to be repeated.

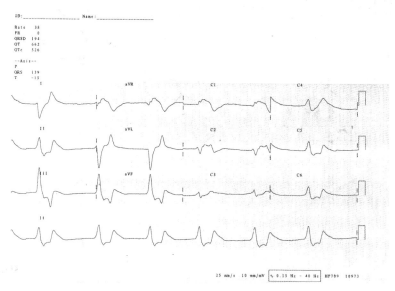

Figure 54.1

An arterial blood gas should be done to determine whether a metabolic acidosis is present. A chest X-ray can help to spot pulmonary oedema.

If acidosis, pulmonary oedema, refractory hyperkalaemia or uraemia are present, renal replacement therapy is indicated. Renal replacement therapy in the acute setting is generally by continuous venovenous haemofiltration (CVVHF). Other modes include continuous venovenous haemodiafiltration (CVVHDF) and continuous venovenous haemodialysis (CVVHD). CVVHF is preferred to dialysis in most acutely ill patients as they tend to have haemodynamic instability and co-morbidities such as heart failure, which makes tolerating rapid fluid transfers difficult.

Once the underlying cause is removed, the majority of patients with an acute kidney injury will make a good recovery, although many may never recover full renal function. A small minority will require lifelong renal replacement therapy.

KEY POINTS

- Acute renal failure is represented by an acute rise in creatinine and can be caused by several processes. It is essential to diagnose the likely cause and target treatment to this.
- Renal replacement therapy becomes necessary if there is refractory hyperkalaemia, uraemia, pulmonary oedema or acidosis.

History

A 78-year-old man was found unrousable in bed by his daughter and has been brought to the emergency department. He is usually fairly independent, looking after himself and going to the local shops, but he has been unwell for two weeks with a chest infection. His GP prescribed a week's course of an antibiotic but that did not help. He had a cough with yellow sputum and was short of breath. He became increasingly lethargic and drowsy, taking to his bed in the past few days. He has had type 2 diabetes for 15 years and is taking metformin and gliclazide. His other medications include ramipril for hypertension, aspirin for a previous transient ischaemic attack (TIA) and simvastatin. He does not drink alcohol and is an ex-smoker.

Examination

The man's mucous membranes appear dry and he has cool peripheries. His jugular venous pulse (JVP) is not visible and heart sounds are normal. He has inspiratory crackles and bronchial breathing in the right base. His abdominal examination is normal. His reflexes are normal. Pupils are equal and reactive to light. His score on the Glasgow Coma Scale is 8/15 (does not open eyes, localizes to pain, makes incomprehensible sounds). A chest X-ray shows right basal consolidation. An ECG shows sinus tachycardia. Observations: temperature 38°C, blood pressure 98/60 mmHg, heart rate 104/min, respiratory rate 30/min, SaO_2 92 per cent on room air.

INVESTIGATIONS		
		Normal range
White cells	19.0	4–11 × 10^9/L
Neutrophils	16	2–7 × 10^9/L
Haemoglobin	17.0	13–18 g/dL
Platelets	350	150–400 × 10^9/L
Sodium	156	135–145 mmol/L
Potassium	6.1	3.5–5.0 mmol/L
Urea	18	3.0–7.0 mmol/L
Creatinine	210	60–110 µmol/L
Chloride	95	95–105 mmol/L
C-reactive protein	288	<5 mg/L
Bilirubin	15	5–25 µmol/L
Alanine aminotransferase	34	8–55 IU/L
Alkaline phosphatase	79	42–98 IU/L
Albumin	56	35–50 g/L
Glucose	37	3.5–5.5 mmol/L
Arterial blood gas on room air:		
pH	7.31	7.35–7.45
PO_2	8.2	9.3–13.3 kPa
PCO_2	3.4	4.7–6.0 kPa
Lactate	2.2	<2 mmol/L
HCO_3	18	22–26 mmol/L
Urinalysis:		
++++ glucose, + protein, no blood, no nitrites or leucocytes, trace ketones		

Questions
- What is the diagnosis?
- How should this patient be managed?

This man is in a hyperosmolar hyperglycaemic state and is showing signs of rapid deterioration towards unconsciousness.

The hyperosmolar hyperglycaemic state is characterized by severe hyperglycaemia (typically a plasma glucose level >35 mmol/L) and hyperosmolality (serum osmolality >340 mosmol/kg) which can be assessed from 2[Na$^+$] + 2[K$^+$] + [urea] + [glucose]. In this case, the serum osmolality works out to be 379 mosmol/kg. He has a mild metabolic acidosis but significant ketoacidosis is not present (pH >7.3 and only a trace of ketones in the urine). This condition mostly occurs in those with type 2 diabetes, in contrast to diabetic ketoacidosis which occurs in type 1 diabetes. However, the distinction is not absolute and up to a third of cases can present with both elements.

Precipitants of this condition are usually infection (pneumonia and urinary tract infection are the most common). Other acute stressors such as myocardial infarction, cerebrovascular accident and surgery can trigger the condition. Significant dehydration, which accompanies this condition, exacerbates electrolyte abnormalities and can cause acute kidney injury.

In this case it is likely that the patient has a severe community-acquired pneumonia that has precipitated this state.

The approach to any critically ill person should start with ABCDE (airway, breathing, circulation, disability, exposure). Each step should consist of an assessment and appropriate management before moving on to subsequent stages. This approach is a logical way of thinking through and dealing with an acutely ill person. This approach is part of the IMPACT (Ill Medical Patient's Acute Care and Treatment) method that is endorsed by the Federation of the Royal Colleges of Physicians and the Royal College of Anaesthetists.

This man's airway is certainly at risk owing to his low GCS score: 8 or below is an indication that a definitive airway is likely to be needed. An anaesthetist should therefore be present to manage this. In the meantime, basic techniques to keep the airway open (head tilt and chin lift or jaw thrust) with or without airway adjuncts (oropharyngeal or nasopharyngeal airways) can be used. High-flow oxygen (10 L/min) using a mask with reservoir should be administered to deliver maximal percentage of oxygen (with this device about 85 per cent oxygen can be given).

Once the airway is secured and oxygen delivered his breathing can be assessed. He is noted to be tachypnoeic, which is a response to the metabolic acidosis from renal impairment secondary to dehydration and sepsis. Auscultation and chest X-ray showed consolidation at the right base. Saturations are low with a PO_2 of 8.2 kPa on air. He has severe respiratory compromise with type 1 respiratory failure. As well as high-flow oxygen he may need assisted ventilation and is at risk of respiratory arrest.

He is hypotensive and tachycardic and requires urgent intravenous access and immediate fluid resuscitation. A urinary catheter should be inserted to quantify urinary output. Shock is defined as inadequate tissue perfusion and several parameters can indicate this (e.g. renal dysfunction, rise in lactate, consciousness level). Shock is likely to be caused by hypovolaemia from fluid depletion and sepsis. An ECG does not show signs of myocardial ischaemia and his JVP is not visible without signs of pulmonary oedema, so cardiogenic shock is unlikely. The initial management is the same. Upon intravenous access a fluid challenge should be given: 250 mL of normal saline should be given over 2 minutes. Response should be checked at 5 minutes. He is likely to be severely dehydrated and will require large volumes of fluid replacement. However, care must be taken in replacing fluid as he is elderly. In general, the first 2 L of normal saline can be given over the first 2 hours. He may require additional colloid boluses if he becomes hypotensive. Subsequently care over aggressive fluid resuscitation is required. Sodium should be reduced slowly and not more than about 10 mmol/L in 24 hours. Further fluid type and duration of administration should be gauged on renal and electrolyte profiles and the patient's haemodynamic status. A central venous line would be helpful to assess central venous pressure in those at risk of heart failure.

Initial observations showed a temperature of 38°C, tachycardia, tachypnoea, and a raised white cell count. He also has evidence of organ failure (renal and neurological). He has all the features of a severe systemic inflammatory response syndrome. It is likely the cause is pneumonia based on the symptoms and signs present. A urine dip did not show evidence of infection, but he should have blood and urine cultures. The combination of hypovolaemic and septic shock is unlikely to respond to fluid resuscitation alone and he will need vasopressor support if he remains hypotensive. Septic shock is associated with a high mortality, up to 50 per cent in some cases. Multi-organ failure is a poor prognostic sign.

In addition to fluids, once sepsis is recognized he should be given antibiotics urgently within the first hour of recognition as advocated by the surviving sepsis campaign (http:// www.survivingsepsis.org). Antibiotics should ideally be targeted to the underlying source, but broad-spectrum organism cover should be initiated without delay.

Serum glucose is corrected slowly with fluid resuscitation and an insulin sliding scale. Potassium levels should be checked every hour in the first 4 hours during fluid resuscitation, as they are likely to decrease as the acidosis improves and the intravascular volume increases.

Renal failure may be exacerbated by underlying diabetes and hypertension, as well as metformin and ramipril. Renal function and hyperkalaemia may improve with fluid resuscitation alone, but renal replacement therapy may be required.

The hyperosmolar hyperglycaemic state is a hypercoagulable condition and thromboprophylaxis is required.

Recognizing that this patient is critically ill is based on the ABCDE approach. Most of the initial management can be instituted in the acute setting, including intubation and invasive monitoring. Once the patient is stable enough he should be transferred to the intensive-care unit for continued management.

 KEY POINTS

- Hyperosmolar hyperglycaemic state is a serious complication that occurs most commonly in elderly people with type 2 diabetes.
- A common trigger for this is infection.
- Coma is rare but is more likely in those presenting with hypernatraemia.

History

A 29-year-old woman has been brought to the emergency department by her husband. He is worried that she is unwell and has been getting worse over the last few days. She describes feeling her heart beating rapidly, difficulty catching her breath, feeling very anxious, hot, sweating a lot, generally weak and confused. She had varicose vein surgery five days ago but had not gone back to work as a schoolteacher because of her symptoms. She was diagnosed with hyperthyroidism secondary to Graves' disease six months ago. She was on carbimazole but stopped taking it a week before her surgery as she was getting a rash. She is taking no other medications. She does not smoke nor drink alcohol.

Examination

This young woman is agitated. She feels warm to the touch and has a bounding regular pulse. She appears mildly dehydrated. Her jugular venous pulse (JVP) is low and there is an ejection systolic murmur over the apex. Respiratory, abdominal and neurological examinations are unremarkable. She is mildly disorientated in time and place. An ECG shows a sinus tachycardia and a chest X-ray has no abnormal features. Observations: temperature 39.0°C, blood pressure 178/85 mmHg, heart rate 110/min, respiratory rate 24/min, SaO_2 98 per cent on room air.

INVESTIGATIONS		
		Normal range
White cells	5.1	$4-11 \times 10^9$/L
Haemoglobin	11.9	13–18 g/dL
Platelets	340	$150-400 \times 10^9$/L
Sodium	142	135–145 mmol/L
Potassium	4.3	3.5–5.0 mmol/L
Urea	7	3.0–7.0 mmol/L
Creatinine	92	60–110 µmol/L
Thyroid-stimulating hormone	Undetectable	0.4–4.0 mIU/L
Free T4	6.7	0.8–1.5 ng/dL
Free T3	310	0.2–0.5 ng/dL

Questions

- What is the most likely diagnosis?
- What should be this patient's immediate management?

ANSWER 56

This woman presents with symptoms and signs characterisitic of a thyroid storm. Thyroid storm is an extreme form of thyrotoxicosis. Thyrotoxicosis is defined as the presence of excessive thyroid hormone from any cause (Graves' disease, toxic multinodular goitre, drug side-effects, excessive thyroid replacement). At which point thyrotoxicosis becomes a thyroid storm can be based on criteria such as those devised by Burch and Wartofsky (see Table 56.1). Criteria are based on the presence of thermoregulatory dysfunction, central nervous system effects, gastrointestinal or hepatic dysfunction and presence of cardiovascular signs. On this scale a score of 45 or greater is highly suggestive of a thyroid storm.

Thyroid storms are a rare presentation; generally milder forms of thyrotoxicosis are more common. Thyroid storms can be triggered in those with a background of hyperthyroidism who have been exposed to stressors such as surgery, severe infection, trauma, myocardial infarction or pregnancy. It can also occur if an antithyroid drug is discontinued. This patient had a diagnosis of Graves' disease and had been on carbimazole but had stopped it due to side-effects. Her recent surgery precipitated thyroid hormone release, which gave rise to her symptoms.

Thyroid storm is life-threatening as patients can develop seizures, coma or heart failure. The goal of treatment is to stop thyroid hormone production and limit its peripheral effects. Initial management starts with an assessment of the patient using the ABCDE approach. In this case she does meet Burch and Watofsksy criteria for a thyroid storm; however, in reality, whether she has thyrotoxicosis or storm the medical management will probably be similar. It should start with supportive therapy including intravenous fluids as she is clinically dehydrated. Pyrexia will cause further dehydration, so paracetamol or other cooling measures can be given to manage her temperature. Urgent administration of propyl-thiouracil to stop production of new hormone and stop the conversion of T4 to T3 should be given. In order to reduce the risk of conversion to thyroid hormone, potassium iodide or Lugol's solution is given after approximately one hour of the initial thiouracil. This blocks further release of hormone from the thyroid gland. A beta-blocker should also be given to counter the effects on the cardiovascular system (propranolol or metoprolol).

Table 56.1 Scoring system due to Burch and Wartofsky (1993)

Diagnostic parameters	Scoring points
Thermoregulatory dysfunction	
Temperature (°C)	
37.2–37.7	5
37.8–38.2	10
38.3–38.8	15
38.9–39.2	20
39.3–39.9	25
>= 40.0	30
Central nervous system effects	
Absent	0
Mild (agitation)	10
Moderate (delirium, psychosis, extreme lethargy)	20
Severe (seizures, coma)	30
Gastrointestinal–hepatic dysfunction	
Absent	0
Moderate (diarrhoea, nausea/vomiting, abdominal pain)	10
Severe (unexplained jaundice)	20
Cardiovascular dysfunction	
Tachycardia (beats/min)	
90–109	5
110–119	10
120–129	15
>= 140	25
Congestive heart failure	
Absent	0
Mild (pedal oedema)	5
Moderate (bibasilar rales)	10
Severe (pulmonary oedema)	15
Atrial fibrillation	
Absent	0
Present	10
Precipitating event	
Absent	0
Present	10

Scoring system: A score of 45 or greater is highly suggestive of thyroid storm; a score of 25–44 is suggestive of impending storm; and a score below 25 is unlikely to represent thyroid storm. Adapted from Burch, Wartofsky L (1993) Life-threatening thyrotoxicosis: thyroid storm, *Endrocrinol Metab Clin North Am* **22**: 263–77 with permission.

 KEY POINTS

- Graves' disease is the most common cause of hyperthyroidism.
- A thyroid storm is an extreme presentation of thyrotoxicosis and is life-threatening if not diagnosed and treated appropriately.

History

A 24-year-old woman attended her GP surgery complaining of severe bouts of headaches that have come and gone over several months. She describes the headaches as pounding. During an attack she feels anxious with palpitations and sweatiness. These episodes can last up to 20 minutes. There is no vomiting, visual disturbance or other neurological symptoms. She feels well between episodes and has no other medical problems. She has tried taking paracetamol and ibuprofen for the headaches but these did not seem to work. She does not drink alcohol nor smoke. There are no significant illnesses in her family history.

Examination

A urinalysis did not show any abnormalities. She appeared sweaty and pale but there was no tremor or evidence of weight loss. Fundoscopy did not show papilloedema or other hypertensive changes. Her heart rate was 120/min and regular, blood pressure 220/110 mmHg and respiratory rate 22/min.

On arrival in the ward her blood pressure is now 190/98 mmHg, heart rate 98/min in sinus rhythm. She appears anxious and her headache is still present. Her cardiorespiratory, abdominal and neurological examinations are all unremarkable. An ECG shows evidence of left ventricular hypertrophy. A chest X-ray is normal.

INVESTIGATIONS		
		Normal range
White cells	6.1	$4–11 \times 10^9$/L
Haemoglobin	12.1	13–18 g/dL
Platelets	260	$150–400 \times 10^9$/L
Sodium	148	135–145 mmol/L
Potassium	4.8	3.5–5.0 mmol/L
Urea	5.4	3.0–7.0 mmol/L
Creatinine	78	60–110 µmol/L
Thyroid-stimulating hormone	2.4 nmol/L	0.4–4.0 mIU/L

Questions
- What is the likely diagnosis and how could it be confirmed?
- What would be appropriate management?

This patient describes intermittent episodes of palpitations, sweating and headache associated with hypertension. These features raise the possibility of an underlying phaeochromocytoma. Other diagnoses to consider are hyperthyroidism (may present with tremor and weight loss but her TSH is normal), carcinoid syndrome (also episodic but presents with intense flushing, associated diarrhoea and wheeze may be present), anxiety attacks (diagnosis of exclusion), recreational drugs (amphetamines and cocaine can mimic the features of an episode).

In phaeochromocytoma these symptoms are due to the episodic release of catecholamines from the tumour. Phaeochromocytomas arise predominantly in the chromaffin cells of the adrenal medulla. They produce adrenaline and noradrenaline. Other sites of tumours include chromaffin cells of the autonomic nervous system (paragangliomas). The surge in catecholamines released by these tumours gives rise to the episodic symptoms and signs (headache, sweating, palipitations and pallor). Tumours are most often benign; malignancy is more likely to occur in paragangliomas. Most cases are sporadic but up to a quarter of cases are hereditary and occur in multiple endocrine neoplasia (MEN) types 2A and 2B, von Hippel–Lindau disease and neurofibromatosis type 1.

Diagnosis is best made with a 24-hour urine collection for catecholamines and metanephrines (the breakdown products of catecholamines), preferably just after an episode. Serum metanephrines and normetanephrines can also be measured. If the urine or blood test is positive, further investigation is required to identify the source. Imaging by MRI or CT of the abdomen and pelvis will identify most phaeochromocytomas. However if very small they can be missed. If the suspicion is high despite a negative CT or MRI, iodine-131 MIGB (metaiodobenzylguanidine) scintigraphy can be performed. This will detect a phaeochromocytoma anywhere and is 99 per cent specific.

She presents with hypertension and a headache. Initial assessment should begin with determining any organ involvement that would necessitate immediate action to lower the blood pressure. In cases of suspected phaeochromocytoma who are not in a hypertensive emergency there are specific management considerations that differ from other causes of severe or malignant hypertension. The treatment aim is to block the effects of catecholamines on the heart and peripheral vasculature by blocking alpha- and beta-receptors. The safest method is administering alpha-blockers first. The reason why beta-blockers cannot be administered right away is that the alpha-receptors in the peripheral vasculature will be completely unopposed. This will lead to vasoconstriction and trigger or worsen a hypertensive crisis. It is important to ensure that patients are adequately hydrated, as a sudden drop in peripheral vascular resistance with alpha-blockade will cause severe hypotension! Normal saline or Hartmann's solution can be used. Adequate hydration is determined by assessment of the central venous pressure (CVP), mucous membranes, skin turgor and urine output. Choice of alpha-blocker is either phenoxybenzamine or doxazosin. Once an alpha-blocker is commenced a beta-blocker such as metoprolol can be administered. The beta-blocker will also reduce the tachycardic effect of catecholamines. If hypertension is not controlled with alpha- and beta-blockade a calcium-channel antagonist can be added. In a hypertensive emergency the first-line treatment of choice should be intravenous phentolamine (alpha-blocker). Nitroprusside infusion is an alternative.

Once blood pressure is controlled surgery should be considered. Recurrence is more likely in those with a hereditary cause. If the tumour is benign then surgery has a high cure rate. Malignant tumours have a variable course depending on timing of diagnosis and treatment modalities.

 KEY POINTS

- Hypertension secondary to phaeochromocytomas should be controlled with the initiation of an alpha-blocker followed by a beta-blocker.
- Hypertension secondary to phaeochromocytomas is rare. However, in young people presenting with hypertension it should be considered as a cause.

History

A 58-year-old man has been brought by ambulance to the emergency department. He returned home three days ago from visiting family members abroad. He started to feel unwell on the flight and was aware of several cases of people with similar symptoms in the city he had been visiting. An outbreak of severe acute respiratory syndrome (SARS) was rumoured, so he moved to stay elsewhere in the country. He returned home a week after moving from the city. He is now unwell with increasing difficulty in breathing and drowsiness. Symptoms started two days ago with myalgia, shortness of breath, cough, headache and chills. He has no existing medical problems and is not on regular medications. He does not smoke or drink alcohol.

Examination

This man appears unwell with shallow respiratory effort. He has reduced chest wall expansion bilaterally. On auscultation there is reduced air entry bilaterally and inspiratory crackles. The jugular venous pulse (JVP) is not elevated and heart sounds are normal. His pulse is thready and rapid and he has cool hands and feet. Abdominal examination is normal. His score on the Glasgow Coma Scale is 14/15 (opens eyes in response to voice, orientated, obeying commands). A chest X-ray is obtained (Fig. 58.1). An ECG reveals sinus tachycardia. Observations: temperature 38.5°C, heart rate 105/min, blood pressure 85/51 mmHg, respiratory rate 28/min, SaO_2 89 per cent on room air.

INVESTIGATIONS		
		Normal range
White cells	12.0	$4–11 \times 10^9$/L
Haemoglobin	11.5	13–18 g/dL
Platelets	376	$150–400 \times 10^9$/L
Sodium	139	135–145 mmol/L
Potassium	3.9	3.5–5.0 mmol/L
Urea	6.0	3.0–7.0 mmol/L
Creatinine	82	60–110 µmol/L
C-reactive protein	98	<5 mg/L
Arterial blood gas on room air:		
pH	7.34	7.35–7.45
PO_2	7.2	9.3–13.3 kPa
PCO_2	3.8	4.7–6.0 kPa
Lactate	2.8	<2 mmol/L
HCO_3	21	22–26 mmol/L

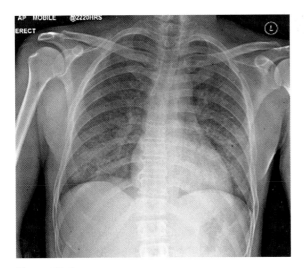

Figure 58.1

Questions
- Give a differential diagnosis for this presentation.
- What should be the immediate management?

ANSWER 58

This returning traveller has presented with sudden onset of respiratory symptoms and signs, having had recent contact with suspected SARS cases. So SARS is indeed a top differential diagnosis. However, other conditions can present in this way. A severe community-acquired pneumonia, atypical pneumonia (*Legionella*, *Chlamydia*, mycoplasma or *Coxiella*), influenza (including the recent pandemic-causing influenza strain influenza A (H1N1), swine influenza, or potentially the H5N1 subtype, avian influenza) can all present in this way and are difficult to tell apart without further investigations. However, the history of preceding events will narrow down the likely causes. His chest X-ray shows bilateral diffuse airspace shadowing.

Severe acute respiratory syndrome was first identified in China in November 2002. In February 2003, SARS was identified as the cause of a sudden outbreak of a respiratory illness that caused high fever, dry cough, myalgia and a sore throat. It started in South East Asia and spread to several countries around the world due to global transmission via travel. It was rapidly progressive with many cases requiring ventilatory support within a week of symptoms first developing. Mortality rate was high, around 10 per cent. The epidemic came to an end in July 2003. The causative organism was a coronavirus. It is suspected to have originated in animals, but the natural reservoir is not known. Sporadic outbreaks have occurred since then but none has developed into an epidemic.

The SARS-coronavirus causes an inflammatory pneumonitis followed by pulmonary fibrosis. Confirmatory tests rely on polymerase chain reaction (PCR) of the viral DNA taken from aspirates or swabs of the nasopharynx. PCR can also be performed on blood and stool specimens. PCR can also rule out other viral causes of an acute respiratory distress syndrome. Changes in blood tests that can occur (leucopenia, elevation of transaminases) also occur in atypical pneumonias and other viral causes. Blood and sputum cultures, serological tests on urine and blood will help to exclude other diagnoses. High-resolution CT of the thorax can show ground-glass opacities and interlobular septal thickening in the majority of SARS cases even with a normal chest X-ray. However, these changes can occur with influenza pneumonitis.

Immediate management of any critically ill patient is the rapid assessment and management of the airway, breathing and circulation (the ABCDE approach to the critically ill person). Regardless of cause, the initial management is the same for anyone presenting in acute respiratory distress. An assessment of airway and breathing indicate he has respiratory failure. He will require intubation and mechanical ventilation as he is at high risk of respiratory arrest. An anaesthetist should be called to assist in airway maintenance. The intensive-care unit should also be notified. In previous outbreaks of SARS about a quarter required ventilation, either non-invasive or invasive. Assessment of his circulation and presence of lactaemia indicate he is shocked. This may be a combination of sepsis and hypovolaemia (a fluid challenge should be administered).

The target should be to preserve organ function. Generally several parameters can help indicate adequate provision of tissue perfusion: CVP 8–12 cmH$_2$O, mean arterial pressure 65 mmHg or more, urine output 0.5 mL/kg per hour, central venous oxygen saturations of 70 per cent or more. Vasopressors are indicated if blood pressure response is refractory after initial fluid resuscitation. Additional supportive care consists of stress ulcer and deep vein thrombosis prophylaxis, blood sugar control, nutritional support, maintaining optimal haemoglobin levels and electrolyte balance.

Current advice from the World Health Organization is that there is no proven treatment for SARS in addition to supportive therapies. However, there may be a role for ribavirin or protease inhibitors (lopinavir or ritonavir) with steroids in severe cases, but there is no formal recommendation for the use of antivirals.

KEY POINTS

- Acute respiratory distress, regardless of infective cause, is managed in the same way initially (support of airway and breathing).
- There is no proven treatment for SARS.
- Suspected cases should be isolated and notified to the Health Protection Agency.

CASE 59: A FATIGUED COLLEGE GIRL

History

A 17-year-old student has been brought to the emergency department after her mother found her in bed drowsy and unable to get up unaided. She is fatigued but does not complain of any paticular problems. However, her mother reports that she has had problems with eating for the past year: she has become a vegetarian and eats only small amounts. Her mother puts this down to stress as the girl is a high-achiever and a perfectionist trying to do many activities at college. She has been very sporty and exercises daily. Lately she has been feeling unwell, generally tired and dizzy but managing to go to college.

Examination

This girl's score on the Glasgow Coma Scale is 14/15 (opening eyes to command, moving limbs spontaneously, coherent speech). She looks very thin, with prominent bony structures (while claiming to be a little overweight) and fine body hair. She has had amenorrhoea for six months. She is not taking any medications and does not smoke or drink alcohol. An ECG demonstrates a sinus bradycardia. Observations: tympanic temperature 36°C, heart rate 40/min, blood pressure 90/60 mmHg.

INVESTIGATIONS		
		Normal range
White cells	6.0	4–11 × 10⁹/L
Haemoglobin	10.5	13–18 g/dL
Platelets	170	150–400 × 10⁹/L
Sodium	128	135–145 mmol/L
Potassium	3.0	3.5–5.0 mmol/L
Urea	5	3.0–7.0 mmol/L
Creatinine	30	60–110 µmol/L
Bilirubin	8	5–25 µmol/L
Alanine aminotransferase	48	8–55 IU/L
Alkaline phosphatase	82	42–98 IU/L
Albumin	30	35–50 g/L
Corrected calcium	2.0	2.2–2.6 mmol/L
Phosphate	0.6	0.8–1.4 mmol/L
Magnesium	0.5	0.6–0.82 mmol/L

Questions:

- What is the diagnosis?
- What would be your immediate management plan?

ANSWER 59

This girl has anorexia nervosa. This is a psychiatric diagnosis characterized by a refusal to maintain normal weight for age and height, a fear of gaining weight, body image distortion and amenorrhoea. There are other subtypes, which include 'restricting' calorie intake, or 'binge eating/purging' behaviours which can include laxative, diuretic or enema use.

She has evidence of a low bodyweight (formal diagnosis relies on an ideal body weight <85 per cent, body mass index <17.5 kg/m²). Her body image perception is altered. She has changed her diet and has been exercising daily. She also has amenorrhoea.

Most people with anorexia nervosa are female, with the onset highest during late adolescence. There is a tendency for other mood disorders and obsessive–compulsive behaviour traits to manifest. The exact cause of anorexia nervosa is not known, but it is thought to have a genetic basis as well as environmental and other social influences.

A heart rate of 40/min and blood pressure of 90/60 mmHg indicate she is haemodynamically unstable. Her electrolyte abnormalities show a metabolic acidosis with hyponatraemia, hypocalcaemia, hypomagnesaemia and hypophosphataemia. She therefore requires high-dependency care with emphasis placed on haemodynamic stability and re-feeding to correct her electrolyte abnormalities.

Her underlying mental status may make re-feeding a difficult task. The main choices are between enteral and parenteral nutrition. Nasogastric feeding is the first method of choice, but this can potentially precipitate re-feeding syndrome. This syndrome is more likely to occur in conditions of electrolyte imbalance and is due to fluid shifts causing delirium, respiratory or cardiac failure as well as gastric dilatation making feeding even more difficult. Other potential complications are progressive neuromuscular dysfunction and prolonging of the QT interval. Thus re-feeding must be done carefully with close observation and monitoring of electrolytes and clinical condition. A dietitian is essential to determine the amount of calories per day as well as supplementation of vitamins and minerals.

Her electrolyte pattern of metabolic acidosis with hypokalaemia could be from purging or laxative abuse. If life-threatening arrhythmias are present from low potassium, then more concentrated amounts can be given, but this would be through a central venous line. Magnesium and calcium levels often need to be corrected before potassium levels become normal. She is also mildly hyponatraemic, which requires correction. It is most likely the result of hypovolaemic hyponatraemia, in which case a 12-hourly bag of 0.9% NaCl would be an acceptable replacement. Beware that sudden changes in sodium levels can precipitate cerebral oedema, seizures and central pontine myelinolysis, so careful replacement must be emphasized depending on the chronicity and severity of hyponatraemia.

Regular monitoring of electrolytes, cardiac arrhythmias and compliance with feeding is best done in a high-dependency unit initially. She should also receive psychiatric support once she is medically stable. Involvement of psychiatric services can also help with re-feeding concerns, as there is potential for patients to be non-compliant with feeding. This is an ethical area and close liaison with psychiatric and medical teams is essential to manage a patient with life-threatening complications of anorexia nervosa.

History

A 25-year-old Caucasian man visited his GP complaining of pain in his lower back and passing red blood in his urine. He had no dysuria or fever. He is generally fit and well, working as a mechanic. He takes no regular medications and has no significant medical history. He does not smoke or drink alcohol. There is no family history of relevance. His only other complaint was of cold-like (coryzal) symptoms for the past few days.

Examination

There were no significant findings by the GP. His blood pressure was 125/65 mmHg. A urine dipstick in the surgery did demonstrate haematuria and trace protein. In view of his symptoms of flank pain and haematuria he was admitted to hospital under the urology team. He underwent a CT scan of his kidneys, ureters and bladder, which did not identify a cause. He was observed for two days as an inpatient; his flank pain settled with analgesia, with improvement in the haematuria.

INVESTIGATIONS		
		Normal range
White cells	5.0	$4–11 \times 10^9$/L
Haemoglobin	15.0	13–18 g/dL
Platelets	250	$150–400 \times 10^9$/L
Sodium	138	135–145 mmol/L
Potassium	4.0	3.5–5.0 mmol/L
Urea	6.5	3.0–7.0 mmol/L
Creatinine	75	60–110 µmol/L
Urine microscopy:		
Numerous red blood cells, no red cell casts, no organisms seen		

Questions:

- What is the most likely diagnosis?
- What are the potential immediate problems that might occur, and how would you manage them?
- How should this patient be followed up?

ANSWER 60

The key findings here are frank haematuria and flank pain. There was no previous history of illness or dysuria, or systemic features. Of note, he appears to have had a recent upper respiratory tract infection. Initial investigation of his urine confirmed haematuria but no infection. No obvious lesion was identified on CT imaging. His observations and blood chemistry were also normal. His condition remained stable and resolved.

The most likely diagnosis with his presenting features is IgA nephropathy. Other differentials to consider are post-streptococcal glomerulonephritis and Henoch–Schönlein purpura.

IgA nephropathy is the most common glomerular disease worldwide. It occurs most commonly in those of Asian or Caucasian origin and is more common in males (2:1). Most cases occur between the ages of 20 and 30. Most cases are sporadic and the cause is not identified, but it tends to occur following an upper respiratory tract infection or gastrointestinal infection.

IgA nephropathy is caused by the deposition of IgA in the glomerular mesangium. Sometimes IgG and complement can also deposit on the mesangium and this is associated with more severe disease. Diagnosis can only be confirmed by renal biopsy and microscopy.

Cases can present in several ways. About half of all cases present as in this case with frank haematuria and flank pain after an upper respiratory tract infection. A third of patients can present with asymptomatic microscopic haematuria. Ten per cent of patients can present with a more severe process characterized by either the nephrotic syndrome or an acute rapidly progressive glomerulonephritis (oedema, hypertension, haematuria and renal failure).

In this case his symptoms were limited and transient. No complicating features were noted. Systemic features are common and include fever, malaise and myalgia.

A urine dipstick test for proteinuria should be performed to identify cases of nephrotic syndrome or acute rapidly progressive glomerulonephritis. Blood pressure should also be checked as a potential presentation is malignant hypertension.

A full renal profile should be checked to rule out renal failure (raised creatinine and urea, hyperkalaemia, metabolic acidosis). Other blood/serological tests should be performed to rule out other causes of glomerular disease, including complement C3 and C4, anti-GBM (glomerular basement membrane), ANCA (antinuclear cytoplasmic antibodies), ANA (antinuclear antibodies), hepatitis virology and HIV.

If the course of the illness is progressive or severe (e.g. renal failure or persistent haematuria/proteinuria) a renal biopsy is required. Findings to support a diagnosis are mesangial deposition of IgA with or without C3.

Cases of persistent proteinuria (with or without hypertension) should be treated with an angiotensin-converting enzyme (ACE) inhibitor or an angiotensin receptor blocker (ARB). These drugs reduce the amount of proteinuria but their role in preventing renal dysfunction is not established.

If a renal biopsy shows changes in keeping with active inflammation, or there is persistent haematuria, there is a role for corticosteroids. A prolonged course (6–12 months or more) may be required.

With more severe disease on biopsy and rapid deterioration in renal function, combined immunosuppressive therapy is indicated (e.g. prednisolone with cyclophosphamide or azathioprine). In crescentic glomerulonephritis, pulsed intravenous methylprednisolone followed by oral prednisolone and cyclophosphamide is used. Plasmapheresis is another alternative but its use is not commonplace. In some cases of acute renal failure, renal replacement therapy may have to be instituted.

The patient in this case should undergo specialist follow-up. Urinalysis, renal function and blood pressure should be checked six-monthly. As his case is mild and self-resolved he does not need long-term follow-up unless there is recurrence with or without progressive symptoms and signs, development of renal failure or hypertension.

 KEY POINTS

- IgA nephropathy is the most common glomerular disease worldwide.
- It can present asymptomatically or with acute renal failure, haematuria, hypertension and oedema.
- Definitive diagnosis is by renal biopsy, but most cases do not require this unless there is significant proteinuria, persistent haematuria or renal impairment.

CASE 61: BRADYCARDIA AND MALAISE

History

A 74-year-old man has been referred to the emergency department following an assessment by his GP, who found him to be unable to get out of his chair and with a slow heart rate of 30/min. He has had a bout of diarrhoea and vomiting over the past couple of days.

Examination

On arrival an ECG is performed (Fig. 61.1). A chest X-ray shows cardiomegaly but clear lung fields. His jugular venous pulse (JVP) is visible 3 cm above the sternal angle with occasional cannon waves. He has dry mucous membranes. He has a midline sternotomy scar. The apex beat is displaced and the impulse diffuse. Heart sounds show a soft pansystolic murmur at the apex. On chest auscultation there are no crackles. Abdominal examination is normal. His ankles are not swollen. He cannot lift his legs off the bed and is generally weak. He has ischaemic heart disease, having had a coronary artery bypass graft one year ago. His other medical history is hypertension, hypercholesterolaemia, type 2 diabetes, gout, benign prostatic hyperplasia (BPH) and congestive heart failure. He has had no chest pains over the last year, although his exercise tolerance is limited to 40 metres on the flat and he has difficulty going up a flight of stairs due to breathlessness. He lives on his own in a flat, mobilizing with a frame. He is on aspirin, bisoprolol, ramipril, spironolactone, bumetanide, atorvastatin, omeprazole, metformin and allopurinol. He has no allergies. He does not smoke or drink alcohol. Observations: temperature 36.4°C, blood pressure 156/78 mmHg, respiratory rate 18/min, SaO_2 94 per cent on room air.

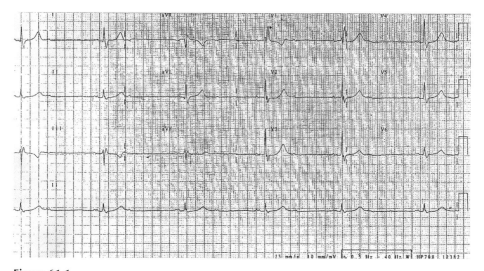

Figure 61.1

		Normal range
White cells	10.0	$4–11 \times 10^9$/L
Haemoglobin	13.3	13–18 g/dL
Platelets	199	$150–400 \times 10^9$/L
Sodium	145	135–145 mmol/L
Potassium	7.9	3.5–5.0 mmol/L
Urea	32	3.0–7.0 mmol/L
Creatinine	245	60–110 µmol/L
Venous blood gas pH	7.35	7.35–7.45

Questions

- What is the main life-threatening abnormality, given the biochemistry and ECG findings?
- What are the potential causes of this?
- How should this patient be further investigated and treated?

ANSWER 61

The main blood abnormality is hyperkalaemia. The level of 7.9 mmol/L is very high and this is the likely cause of his muscle weakness and complete heart block (shown on the ECG and indicated clinically by the bradycardia and cannon waves). He also has renal impairment.

Hyperkalaemia has several causes, so focusing investigations is crucial to allow timely and appropriate treatment. Often a combination of underlying problems may be the cause. In this case the most important to consider are:

- worsening chronic kidney disease;
- drug-related;
- obstruction;
- cardio-renal syndrome;
- volume depletion.

Urgent investigations should include a renal ultrasound scan to look for obstruction causing hydronephrosis. It will also help to assess renal size and give an indication as to whether there is likely to be pre-existing chronic renal impairment. A venous blood gas will show if there is metabolic acidosis. Although he has congestive heart failure he has no signs of it at present. He is likely to be dehydrated from the recent diarrhoea and vomiting.

He is on multiple medications that can cause hyperkalaemia directly or indirectly. Spironolactone is a potassium-sparing diuretic and can raise potassium in some people who are sensitive to this drug. Ramipril can cause hyperkalaemia and in states of volume depletion from recent diarrhoea and vomiting this is exacerbated. Bumetanide, a loop diuretic, will exacerbate volume depletion but tend to lower serum potassium. Heart failure is linked to renal impairment: the relationship is complex and it is known that one exacerbates the other. This phenomenon is termed cardio-renal syndrome.

Management should be based on the immediate need to lower his potassium level and treat his complete heart block. An assessment should be made of haemodynamic stability. If he shows signs of hypotension or heart failure or reduced consciousness, he should be given atropine 500 µg intravenously to try to increase the heart rate. Further doses can be administered to a maximum of 3 mg. Isoprenaline infusion is a useful drug to use. If these measures do not work he will need initiation of transcutaneous pacing with a view to inserting a temporary pacing wire.

Ten per cent calcium chloride or gluconate should be given intravenously as soon as possible. Calcium works by stabilizing the cardiac sarcolemmal membrane, but its effects wear off in minutes so repeated doses may be necessary. Intravenous insulin/dextrose should be commenced to drive the potassium into cells; repeated doses are often required. He is clinically dehydrated and fluid resuscitation should also be administered; normal saline is an appropriate fluid. A fluid challenge can be administered to determine the effect on blood pressure and urine output. He has a history of congestive cardiac failure, so careful fluid resuscitation is important. To help assess fluid balance, a central venous line may be required. He should be admitted to the intensive-care unit or coronary unit for continuous cardiac monitoring. If potassium is not improving with insulin/dextrose and fluid resuscitation, he requires renal replacement therapy.

Once potassium levels start to come down his rhythm may return to normal. Also his renal function should improve with fluids as this episode is likely to have been precipitated by dehydration from a recent illness made worse by medications. Metformin, aspirin and allopurinol should all be discontinued in the short term. Metformin is associated with lactic acidosis in the setting of significant renal failure.

Significant hyperkalaemia is defined as K >6 mmol/L, while moderate hyperkalaemia is 5–6 mmol/L; all levels above 6 should be treated. Treatment should be given between 5 and 6 if associated with ECG changes. ECG changes in hyperkalaemia include early changes (peaked T waves, shortening of the QT interval and ST segment depression). Later changes are widening of the QRS complex, prolongation of the PR interval and eventual loss of P waves. Eventually the QRS complex widens further to appear as a sine wave. At this point ventricular fibrillation or asystole can follow. However, any arrhythmia can be caused, including various degrees of AV block.

 KEY POINTS

- Hyperkalaemia is life-threatening. When found, an ECG must be performed in all cases.
- Hyperkalaemia has many causes and the diagnosis is based on a focused history, examination and appropriate investigations.

CASE 62: BLEEDING GUMS AND NOSE

History

A 58-year-old man has presented to the emergency department with a nose-bleed and bleeding gums, which have continued for nearly 24 hours. He also has a fever, cough and shortness of breath which appeared over the past few days. Prior to this he had been fairly well. He has a medical history of hypertension, hypercholesterolaemia, psoriasis and osteoarthritis of the hips. He has taken methotrexate for his psoriasis for two years, as well as omeprazole, bendroflumethiazide, ramipril and paracetamol. He has no allergies. He does not smoke or drink alcohol.

Examination

This man is alert and oriented. He has active bleeding of his gums and ongoing epistaxis. There is bruising over his arms and legs. Cardiovascular, neurological and abdominal examinations are unremarkable. On respiratory examination there is reduced air entry at the left base with inspiratory crackles, and a chest X-ray shows left basal consolidation. No lymphadenopathy is found. An ECG shows a sinus tachycardia. Observations: temperature 38.2°C, blood pressure 110/78 mmHg, heart rate 101/min, respiratory rate 24/min, SaO_2 94 per cent on room air.

INVESTIGATIONS		
		Normal range
White cells	2.1	$4–11 \times 10^9$/L
Neutrophils	0.9	$2–7 \times 10^9$/L
Lymphocytes	0.6	$1–4 \times 10^9$/L
Monocytes	0.2	$0.2–0.8 \times 10^9$/L
Basophils	32	$40–900 \times 10^6$/L
Eosinophils	0.12	$0.04–0.44 \times 10^9$/L
Haemoglobin	9.5	13–18 g/dL
Platelets	36	$150–400 \times 10^9$/L
Sodium	142	135–145 mmol/L
Potassium	4.8	3.5–5.0 mmol/L
Urea	7.0	3.0–7.0 mmol/L
Creatinine	131	60–110 µmol/L
C-reactive protein	234	<5 mg/L

Questions:

- What are the main abnormalities on full blood count?
- What could be the cause in this case?
- What should be the management of this patient?

The main abnormalities are a low haemoglobin, low white cell count and low platelet count (pancytopenia). Severe pancytopenia is defined as WCC below 0.5×10^9/L, platelets below 20×10^9/L with an anaemia causing symptoms. He presents with bleeding and bruising as well as signs of sepsis, such as a fever and tachycardia. All components of the white cell count are low. Of particular concern is the low neutrophil count, which will put the patient at increased risk of bacterial infections and, ultimately, neutropenic sepsis.

The mechanisms of pancytopenia are either failure or reduction in haematopoetic bone marrow function by inadequate stem cell function. Stem cell function can be affected by certain drugs, such as methotrexate and chemotherapeutic agents; by infiltration into the bone marrow, which can occur in malignancy and infections such as tuberculosis; and stem cell failure. In some cases pancytopenia results from increased destruction in the circulation or spleen. A combination of mechanisms may also be responsible. The causes of a pancytopenia include:

- infection – viral (HIV, EBV, CMV), brucellosis;
- malignancy – infiltrative (prostate, thyroid, breast, kidney, leukaemia, myeloma, lymphoma, myelodysplasia);
- other bone marrow disorders – myelofibrosis;
- chemotherapy (cytotoxic);
- severe megaloblastic anaemia – vitamin B_{12} deficiency, folic acid deficiency;
- paroxysmal nocturnal haemoglobinuria;
- chronic liver disease;
- drug-induced – sulphonamides, rifampicin, quinine, methotrexate;
- connective tissue diseases (systemic lupus erythematosus, rheumatoid arthritis).

In this case he was relatively well prior to the recent problems. There was no lymphadenopathy, hepatosplenomegaly, or loss of weight, making malignancy less likely. There were no signs of chronic liver disease or connective tissue disease. He is on methotrexate and this may be the cause.

Methotrexate works by inhibiting dihydrofolate reductase. This enzyme converts dihydrofolate to tetrahydrofolate, which is required for nucleoside production and DNA synthesis. Inhibiting the enzyme results in DNA and RNA synthesis inhibition. Thus in rapidly dividing cells methotrexate inhibition of DNA and RNA production results in cell death; hence its use as a cytotoxic chemotherapy agent. In lower doses it is also used to treat autoimmune disorders (rheumatoid arthritis, Crohn's disease, psoriasis). The mechanism of action is thought to involve the modulation of the inflammatory response rather than its effects on purine and pyrimidine synthesis inhibition seen with higher doses. Folic acid supplementation is therefore required for these patient groups. So in methotrexate overdose or lack of folic acid supplementation immunosuppression can occur. There are several case reports that even in lower doses it can cause immunosuppression despite folic acid supplementation; the underlying reasons for this are not clear.

The initial management of this patient involves treating his bleeding, sepsis and pancytopenia. Assessment of his airway, breathing and circulation is crucial to determine his subsequent management. He is stable from this point of view and the focus can move on to addressing the bleeding, sepsis and pancytopenia.

He will need replacement of blood and platelets as he has active bleeding. Tranexamic acid will help clot formation. Clotting should also be checked and any abnormalities should be treated. Liaising with a haematologist is therefore advised. An urgent blood film and bone marrow biospy would most likely be performed in this case to aid diagnosis. Serial monitoring of full blood count is required, with replacement of platelets and haemoglobin as necessary.

Blood culture and sputum culture are important as soon as possible, but start broad-spectrum cover that treats a suspected pneumonia. Once the cultures grow an organism and sensitivities are known, the antibiotics can be adjusted if necessary. This patient has markers of sepsis and this should be treated aggressively especially in the case of immunosupression. Barrier nursing and isolation may be needed if his WCC count drops further.

Control of bleeding can be achieved by the administration of blood products and tranexamic acid. Clotting factors can be replaced if the clotting profile is deranged. However, if epistaxis does not stop he may require intervention.

 KEY POINTS

- Methotrexate can cause myelosupression at low and high doses.
- Pancytopenia can present as sepsis, bleeding or both.

History

A 75-year-old woman presented to her GP with palpitations and exertional shortness of breath. She had been experiencing palpitations intermittently over the last two years but had noticed her heart racing more often. She now gets short of breath when going up stairs. She is taking medications for hypertension. She does not smoke or drink alcohol. She is systemically well and has no other significant medical or family history. As her symptoms were getting worse her GP decided to refer her to the medical admissions unit.

Examination

Her pulse is irregularly irregular with a rate of about 120/min. On cardiovascular and respiratory examination there is a raised jugular venous pressure (JVP), displaced apex beat and fine inspiratory crackles at the lung bases, with mild swelling of her ankles. Her blood pressure is 160/75 mmHg. An ECG is shown in Fig. 63.1 and a chest X-ray in Fig. 63.2. Respiratory rate is normal and her pulse oximetry is also normal. Her heart rate slowed down slightly following initial treatment in the emergency department but the examination findings remained unchanged.

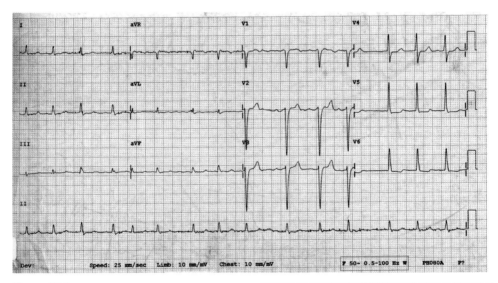

Figure 63.1

Questions

- What is the diagnosis?
- What are the likely causes?
- How should this patient be managed?

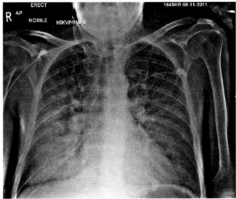

Figure 63.2

ANSWER 63

This woman has atrial fibrillation with a fast ventricular response. The ECG shows atrial fibrillation: note that there are no P waves before the QRS complex, which is narrow, and that the heart rate is irregularly irregular. The fast rate and the loss of atrial transport from the fibrillation will impair cardiac function. The basal inspiratory crackles suggest that she has LV dysfunction. The chest X-ray shows fluffy, interstitial shadowing and prominent upper-lobe blood diversion, suggestive of pulmonary oedema.

Initial management should focus on determining the presence or absence of chest pain, pulmonary oedema and haemodynamic instability. Hypotension or worsening pulmonary oedema is a sign that she is not tolerating the irregular fast ventricular rates and she will then need to be cardioverted either electrically or chemically. However, in this case, although she does have signs of fluid overload, she is haemodynamically stable and comfortable at rest.

Atrial fibrillation becomes more common with increasing age such that more than 10 per cent of those aged over 80 years have AF. The most common causes of AF are hypertension, heart failure, ischaemic heart disease and valvular disease. Hyperthyroidism is another cause and may not have obvious clinical signs in the elderly.

Initial management should focus on managing immediate complications, controlling the ventricular rate and consideration of antithrombotic therapy. She is in mild heart failure (NYHA class 2). According to current evidence and guidance, rate control without rhythm control is a reasonable initial approach. First-line therapy involves beta-blockers or non-dihydropyridine calcium-channel blockers. However, this patient has signs of heart failure on clinical examination and on chest X-ray. Commencing with digoxin may be better in this situation as it is not a negative inotrope. In this case, the patient was loaded with digoxin in the emergency department and then continued on a maintenance dose. She should undergo an echocardiogram to assess LV size and function and any valvular pathology that might underlie her AF.

Concomitantly she should be assessed for stroke risk. Warfarin (or equivalent agent) is preferred as anticoagulation if one or more stroke risk factors are present. Stroke risk can be estimated from a score (CHA$_2$DS$_2$VASc: Congestive heart failure, Hypertension, Age ≥75 (doubled), Diabetes, Stroke (doubled), Vascular disease, Age 65–74, and Sex category (female) – see Table 63.1A). A score of 2 predicts a 2.2 per cent per year adjusted stroke risk (see Table 63.1B). This is generally accepted to be the cut-off to starting treatment with an oral anticoagulant provided there are no contraindications.

Table 63.1A CHA₂DS₂VASc scoring

Table 63.1A CHA$_2$DS$_2$VASc scoring

Risk factor	Score[a]
Congestive heart failure / LV dysfunction	1
Hypertension	1
Age ≥75 years	2
Diabetes mellitus	1
Stroke / transient ischaemic attack / thromboembolism	2
Vascular disease[b]	1
Age 65–74 years	1
Sex category (female sex)	1

[a]Maximum score is 9 (age may contribute 0, 1 or 2 points).
[b]Vascular disease represents prior myocardial infarction, peripheral arterial disease, aortic plaque.
Adapted from 'Guidelines for the management of atrial fibrillation ESC', *Eur Heart J*, 2010, **31**: 2369–429 with permission.

Table 63.1B Adjusted stroke risk according to the CHA$_2$DS$_2$VASc score

Score	Adjusted stroke risk (per year)
0	0%
1	1.3%
2	2.2%
3	3.2%
4	4.0%
5	6.7%
6	9.8%
7	9.6%
8	6.7%
9	5.2%

Adapted from 'Guidelines for the management of atrial fibrillation ESC', *Eur Heart J*, 2010, **31**: 2369–429 with permission.

The main concern with anticoagulants is the risk of bleeding and an assessment of this risk should be made prior to starting treatment. A bleeding risk score such as HAS-BLED can be used to assess risk (see Table 63.2). Warfarin is still the anticoagulant of choice. Direct thrombin inhibitors are likely to be licensed for use in AF.

Table 63.2 HAS-BLED bleeding risk score

Letter	Clinical characteristic	Points awarded
H	Hypertension	1
A	Abnormal renal or liver function (1 point each)	1 or 2
S	Stroke	1
B	Bleeding	1
L	Lable INRs	1
E	Elderly (age >65 years)	1
D	Drugs (NSAIDs and antiplatelets) or alcohol (1 point each)	1 or 2

NSAIDs, non-steroidal anti-inflammatory drugs.
Reproduced from 'Guidelines for the management of atrial fibrillation ESC', *Eur Heart J*, 2010, **31**: 2369–429 with permission.

 KEY POINTS

- Atrial fibrillation, particularly with a fast ventricular response rate, will lead to a reduced ejection fraction and impaired cardiac function.
- Rate control is important, to ensure that the ventricles fill sufficiently, and medications such as beta-blockers and digoxin may be necessary to achieve this.
- Atrial fibrillation causes stasis of blood within the heart chambers, increasing the risk of embolic stroke. Anticoagulation is often commenced to prevent this, but the risk of bleeding with warfarin and heparin needs to be considered.

CASE 64: PETECHIAL RASH AND LOSS OF CONSCIOUSNESS

History

A 28-year-old man with Down's syndrome has been brought to the emergency department after being discovered unconscious in his own home. His parents say that he has been very lethargic lately. Last night he complained of a generalized headache, nausea and vomiting, and blurred vision. This morning his parents found him in bed unrousable.

Examination

This man looks unwell. Shortly after arrival, he had a tonic–clonic seizure which self-terminated in 1 minute. There is a petechial rash, especially on pressure-dependent areas. In the neck there are palpable, tender cervical lymph nodes. In the mouth, gum hypertrophy and small ulcers are noted. Capillary refill is 3 seconds with cold peripheries. The rest of the cardiorespiratory examinations are unremarkable. There is hepatosplenomegaly on abdominal palpation. His Glasgow Coma Scale score is E3/V3/M4. His neck is stiff but there is no focal neurology, with normal tone on peripheral nervous system examination. There is a positive Babinski sign bilaterally. Pupils are equal and reactive to light, but direct ophthalmoscopy is difficult as he is uncooperative. Observations: temperature 38.5°C, heart rate 112/min, respiratory rate 32/min, blood pressure 90/60 mmHg.

INVESTIGATIONS		
		Normal range
White cells	52.0	4–11 × 10^9/L
Haemoglobin	5.0	13–18 g/dL
Platelets	12	150–400 × 10^9/L
Sodium	135	135–145 mmol/L
Potassium	3.5	3.5–5.0 mmol/L
Urea	10	3.0–7.0 mmol/L
Creatinine	180	60–110 µmol/L
C-reactive protein	121	<5 mg/L
Bilirubin	35	5–25 µmol/L
Alanine aminotransferase	70	8–55 IU/L
Alkaline phosphatase	200	42–98 IU/L
Albumin	18	35–50 g/L
INR	1.9	0.9–1.1
D-dimer	5.2	<0.55 mg/L
Fibrinogen	0.7	1.7–3.2 g/L
Blood film: predominantly blast cells		
Arterial blood gas on room air:		
pH	7.30	7.35–7.45
PO_2	10.0	9.3–13.3 kPa
PCO_2	3.0	4.7–6.0 kPa
Lactate	6.0	<2 mmol/L
HCO_3	18	22–26 mmol/L
Base excess	−6	−3 to +3 mmol/L

Questions

- What is the likely unifying diagnosis?
- What should be the initial management plan?

The best diagnosis is menigococcal septicaemia secondary to acute leukaemia. The full blood count has an extremely high white cell count and the blood film comments that the majority of cells are blast cells. This patient almost certainly has acute lymphocytic leukaemia, although a bone marrow sample will be needed to confirm the diagnosis. People with Down's syndrome are genetically predisposed to developing leukaemias.

Despite the high white cell count, the cells are poorly formed and ineffective. Patients with leukaemia are therefore at risk of developing life-threatening infections.

This patient also has a low platelet count and low fibrinogen level, as well as a high INR and D-dimer. These are all features highly suggestive of disseminated intravascular coagulation. Disseminated intravascular coagulation (DIC) can develop in the presence of severe sepsis. The clotting mechanisms are activated and small thrombi form in the blood vessels. These clots consume large numbers of platelets and clotting factors, thus also causing abnormal bleeding. Patients can present with haemorrhage or thromboembolic disease, causing multi-organ failure, and this is a medical emergency. In this case, it seems that the source of the sepsis, precipitating DIC, is likely to be a meningococcal meningitis (neck stiffness and photophobia).

He should be nursed in the recovery position with high-flow oxygen and monitored in a high-dependency area. His glucose should be checked immediately and a neurological examination performed after his seizure. Establish intravenous access if not already done so, and have lorazepam ready if this man begins to have another seizure.

In the clinical context of probable meningococcal septicaemia, one would not need to perform a lumbar puncture to confirm the diagnosis. Instead the focus is on rapidly resuscitating his septic shock and DIC. A referral to intensive care should be considered early whilst resuscitating this man. As a biomarker, high lactate is closely correlated with the need for critical-care admissions and mortality. A recent retrospective analysis suggests that even a 'normal' lactate from above 0.75 is correlated with mortality and poor outcome during a hospital admission.

This man should be resuscitated according to the Surviving Sepsis guidelines (http://www.survivingsepsis.org), with emphasis on early institution of broad-spectrum antimicrobials and goal-directed therapy for ongoing organ support. It is important to obtain blood cultures prior to antibiotic administration, but this should not delay any institution of antibiotic therapy. With his current coagulation disorder it may be difficult to perform invasive procedures such as central venous catheterization and arterial line insertion. High levels of blood products are probably needed to support bone marrow failure and DIC. Ideally, blood products negative for cytomegalovirus (CMV) should be given until his CMV status is known, as he is at risk of CMV viraemia and associated pathology.

The treatment of DIC can be complex as it often occurs in the context of critically unwell patients. Support with blood products forms the mainstay of treatment in DIC (platelets, cryoprecipitate and fresh frozen plasma). Close liaison with a haematologist is advisable. The mortality rate of acute severe DIC is high.

History

A 36-year-old woman has presented with severe shortness of breath associated with wheeze and productive cough. She was diagnosed with asthma at age 10 years. Until a year ago she had never been admitted to hospital, but since then she has been admitted three times with asthma exacerbations. She also complains of a chronic productive cough with large quantities of thick, dark sputum that is hard to expectorate. There is no other medical history, including sinusitis. She has never smoked. There is no travel history. She is taking salbutamol inhaler, 2 puffs four times daily; Seretide 250, 2 puffs twice daily; montelukast, 10 mg once daily; Uniphyllin Continus, 200 mg twice daily.

Examination

This woman looks unwell and has pursed-lip breathing. There is no clubbing or lymphadenopathy, peripheral oedema or rash. Jugular venous pressure (JVP) is not raised. Her chest wall is overexpanded and chest expansion reduced but equal on both sides, and her trachea is central. There are coarse inspiratory crackles bibasally and polyphonic expiratory wheezes throughout her chest. A chest X-ray shows multiple areas of consolidation and thickened bronchial wall markings. Observations: heart rate 120/min, regular and with good volume, respiratory rate 28/min, SaO_2 92 per cent on room air.

INVESTIGATIONS		
		Normal range
White cells	7.0	$4–11 \times 10^9$/L
Neutrophils	5.0	$2–7 \times 10^9$/L
Lymphocytes	0.9	$1–3.5 \times 10^9$/L
Eosinophils	2	$0.04–0.44 \times 10^9$/L
Haemoglobin	12.0	13–18 g/dL
Platelets	188	$150–400 \times 10^9$/L
C-reactive protein	24	<5 mg/L
Urine	Protein 1+ only	
pANCA	Positive	
anti-MPO	Positive	
PEFR	100 L/min	
Arterial blood gas on room air:		
pH	7.48	7.35–7.45
PO_2	7.9	9.3–13.3 kPa
PCO_2	3.2	4.7–6.0 kPa
Lactate	2.0	<2 mmol/L
HCO_3	24	22–26 mmol/L
Base excess	0	−3 to +3 mmol/L

Questions

- What are the differential diagnoses of this patient's clinical deterioration, and how would you confirm the diagnosis?
- What should be the initial management plan?
- What should be the follow-up plan?

ANSWER 65

This woman's chest sounds wheezy and there are coarse crackles throughout. The chest X-ray shows thickened bronchial wall markings and areas of infiltration and consolidation, consistent with chronic inflammation and infection. The patient probably has a degree of underlying bronchiectasis. Bronchiectasis occurs when there is chronic inflammation in the lungs for a long period, leading to permanent dilatation of the aiways. The blood tests show a marked eosinophilia.

There are a number of disorders that cause blood eosinophilia and pulmonary infiltrates on chest radiograph; but with the history of asthma, the two most likely diagnoses are allergic bronchopulmonary aspergillosis (ABPA) and Churg–Strauss syndrome.

ABPA is a condition that occurs when there is an abnormal immune response to *Aspergillus* spores. *Aspergillus* is a fungus that is ubiquitous and is present in the sputum of most people. In ABPA, patients develop a heightened immune response to the spores and the airways become inflamed. There is a long history of chronic inflammation and the bronchiectatic changes arise. Patients present with wheezing due to bronchoconstriction, shortness of breath and mucus plugging, as well as recurrent chest infections.

Churg–Strauss syndrome is a vasculitic disorder of small and medium-sized vessels. The American College of Rheumatology criteria for the classification for Churg–Strauss syndrome require four of the following six criteria to establish the diagnosis:

- asthma;
- blood eosinophilia >10 per cent of total peripheral white cell count;
- mono- or peripheral neuropathy;
- sinus disease;
- extravascular eosinophilic infiltration of tissue biopsy;
- pulmonary infiltrates.

The given history and examination findings do not fit the diagnostic criteria of Churg–Strauss syndrome; and that, together with the lack of evidence of renal involvement, suggests ABPA as the most likely diagnosis here.

It is important to diagnose ABPA to provide effective treatment and reduce the chronic inflammation and remodelling changes occurring in the airways. The diagnosis of ABPA can be established by:

- serum IgG *Aspergillus* precipitins;
- raised total serum IgE;
- skin-prick sensitivity to *Aspergillus*;
- sputum sample demonstrating *Aspergillus* hyphae and eosinophilia.

It is important to review the travel and drug history in eosinophilic lung disorders as other diagnoses should be explored if these are present (e.g. tropical pulmonary eosinophilia, Löffler's syndrome).

The initial management plan should be similar to any patients presenting with an acute severe asthma attack. It is important to assess the severity of the asthma attack and to find out important features in the history, such as 'normal' peak expiratory flow rate and history of intensive care admissions etc. In patients taking aminophylline, a drug serum level should be obtained. Treatment should include high-flow oxgen, bronchodilating nebulizers titrated according to clinical response, steroids and, in some cases, magnesium sulphate infusion.

Given the history of this patient, it is important to establish whether she has bronchiectasis, and this can be confirmed on high-resolution chest CT.

Once the diagnosis of ABPA is established, the mainstay treatment is with oral steroids. The antifungal itraconazole had been previously shown to be helpful in reducing exacerbations of ABPA.

 KEY POINTS

- Worsening asthma symptoms in previously well-controlled asthmatic patients should prompt investigation of the underlying cause.
- Acute asthma attack is a common medical emergency that should be dealt with promptly. National guidelines are available to guide management decisions.

CASE 66: WHEEZE AND SHORTNESS OF BREATH

History
A 38-year-old man has presented to the emergency department with shortness of breath and wheeze. On arrival he was in extremis and unable to complete a full sentence. He was discharged from the hospital one week ago after acute severe exacerbation of chronic obstructive pulmonary disease (COPD), first diagnosed three years ago. This is his third casualty attendance over the past 12 months. He smokes five cigarettes a day. He is now awaiting investigation for deranged liver function tests. His father died of a chest disease in his 30s. He is taking salbutamol inhaler p.r.n.; tiotropium, 18 µg once daily; Symbicort 6/200, 2 puffs daily; carbocisteine, 375 mg thrice daily; Uniphyllin Continus, 400 mg twice daily.

Examination
This man is visibly dyspnoeic with a respiratory rate of 32/min. His trachea is central, expansion of the chest poor but equal, and auscultation reveals widespread expiratory wheeze but no clinical sign of consolidation. A chest X-ray shows hyperinflated lung fields. Observations: heart rate 130/min, blood pressure 130/80 mmHg, SaO_2 91 per cent on FiO_2 0.4.

INVESTIGATIONS		
		Normal range
White cells	15.0	$4–11 \times 10^9$/L
Haemoglobin	13.0	13–18 g/dL
Platelets	150	$150–400 \times 10^9$/L
Sodium	140	135–145 mmol/L
Potassium	3.2	3.5–5.0 mmol/L
Urea	7.1	3.0–7.0 mmol/L
Creatinine	100	60–110 µmol/L
C-reactive protein	10	<5 mg/L
Bilirubin	50	5–25 µmol/L
Aspartate aminotransferase	49	8–40 IU/L
Alkaline phosphatase	600	42–98 IU/L
Albumin	31	35–50 g/L
INR	1.2	0.9–1.1
Arterial blood gas on FiO_2 0.4:		
pH	7.23	7.35–7.45
PO_2	7.8	9.3–13.3 kPa
PCO_2	8.2	4.7–6.0 kPa
Lactate	2.3	<2 mmol/L
HCO_3	29	22–26 mmol/L

Questions
- What are the differential diagnoses?
- What is the appropriate initial management?
- What is the unifying diagnosis and how would you confirm it?

The main differential diagnoses for this man's acute shortness of breath include asthma, acute exacerbation of COPD, pneumonia, and acute pulmonary oedema. Pneumothorax and pulmonary embolism should also be considered but are much less likely.

This man presented with type 2 respiratory acidosis and partially compensated metabolic alkalosis. His arterial blood gas result is worrying and needs urgent action: referral to the critical care service should be considered. As with all acutely unwell patients, airway, breathing and circulation should be managed accordingly and he should be nursed in a high-dependency area, with cardiorespiratory monitoring. Venous access should be established and a 12-lead ECG should be taken. A chest radiograph should be requested to look for acute pulmonary oedema, pneumothorax and pneumonia. In this case, the chest X-ray showed hyperexpanded lung fields.

The definition and treatment of acute exacerbation of COPD is well summarized by the NICE guideline CG12. The pharmacological management includes appropriate oxygen therapy, bronchodilators (β_2 agonists, anticholinergics and theophyllines), steroids and antibiotics.

Oxygen is a drug and it should be given appropriately by selecting an appropriate delivery device. Various types of mask are classified into variable (nasal cannulae, Hudson masks) and fixed-performance (Venturi masks, non-rebreathing reservoir masks, and masks delivering non-invasive ventilation). A fixed-performance device is so called because the fraction of inspired oxygen (FiO_2) is known; it is commonly quoted as FiO_2 or percentage oxygen (e.g. FiO_2 0.4 = 40 per cent oxygen). For variable-performance devices the FiO_2 is unknown, so it is impossible to prescribe FiO_2 0.24 if oxygen is delivered by nasal cannulae; instead one should quote the amount of oxygen in litres delivered (e.g. 4 L oxygen via nasal cannulae). For variable-performance devices, the amount of FiO_2 being received by the patient depends on, for example, the type of device and respiratory rate and tidal volume. A fixed-performance device should be used in patients at risk of type 2 respiratory failure. (Type 1 respiratory failure = PaO_2 <8 kPa; type 2 = PaO_2 <8 kPa and $PaCO_2$ >6.7 kPa.) This may be difficult to predict and the key is to ensure hypoxia is corrected (PaO_2 >8 kPa) and to perform frequent clinical assessment to look for clinical signs of CO_2 narcosis and to perform sequential arterial blood gas sampling to look for interval changes in PaO_2 and $PaCO_2$ values. The usual practice is to perform arterial blood gas sampling 30 minutes after a change of FiO_2 or device (if clinically appropriate). The dose of oxygen should be chosen and titrated according to these results. For patients not at risk of type 2 respiratory failure, it is appropriate to aim for oxygen saturations of >94 per cent (assessed on pulse oximeter and arterial blood gas sampling). For patients at risk of type 2 respiratory failure, it may be appropriate to aim for oxygen saturation of 88–92 per cent, depending on the clinical scenario. Oxygen should be maintained to >8 kPa; below this level the total amount of oxygen available to tissues will be dangerously variable and low as demonstrated by the haemoglobin oxygen dissociation curve.

Non-invasive ventilation in the form of bilevel positive airway pressure (BIPAP), delivered via a face or nasal mask, has revolutionized the management of type 2 respiratory failure in COPD. The British Thoracic Society (BTS) has published a guideline on its use. These patients should be ideally managed in critical-care units where access to mechanical ventilation is rapid. Bronchodilators could be delivered via BIPAP device concurrently which is useful in the treatment of acute exacerbation of COPD.

In acute severe exacerbation of COPD (or asthma), a 'back to back' nebulizers strategy is used. This is mainly for β_2 agonists such as salbutamol. For salbutamol nebulizer it is probably better to prescribe a 2.5 mg rather than 5 mg dose to minimize the adrenergic side-effects. To achieve equivalent bronchodilating effects, the low dose could be given more frequently. Salbutamol should rarely be given above 10 mg per hour. If this is needed, other bronchodilators or ventilation strategies should be considered because, beyond this dose, it may cause excessive tachycardia, peripheral vasodilation, hyperlactataemia and hypokalaemia. In order to achieve appropriate drug delivery, nebulizers should be driven by 8 L of air or oxygen; therefore in patients with type 2 respiratory failure it is important to notify nursing staff to deliver nebulizer therapy through medical air. If oxygen therapy is needed then it could be temporarily delivered via nasal cannulae. Patients taking oral theophylline therapy should have theophylline level measured at admission to determine whether it is subtherapeutic or at toxic level. This is particularly important if intravenous theophylline therapy is considered.

The decision to initiate antibiotics may be difficult at times when there is no sign of focal consolidation. It may be appropriate to initiate antibiotics if there is a change of sputum colour or frequency or clinical signs of sepsis. Steroids should be given in all severe COPD exacerbations.

This man was diagnosed with COPD at a very young age with a minimal smoking history. It may be appropriate to review his case histories and previous lung function tests, chest imaging and bronchodilator reversibility tests to ensure this patient is not suffering from asthma rather than COPD. If COPD is confirmed then further investigation should be considered. In the setting of a positive family history of early death due to chest disease and a history of deranged liver function tests, one should certainly consider α1-antitrypsin deficiency.

α1-Antitrypsin deficiency (A1AD) is a disease which has various phenotypes (designated M, S, ZZ). It is one of the most commonly inherited genetic disorders. MM confers 100 per cent protease inhibitor activity but ZZ is the most severe A1AD phenotype. The severity of lung disease differs even in siblings with the same allele. This is partially explained by environmental factors such as smoking and dust exposure; therefore it is paramount to educate patients with α1-antitrypsin deficiency not to smoke. Presentation (if not diagnosed through family screening) is often at the third or fourth decade with emphysematous lung changes out of proportion to smoking history. The emphysematous changes are predominately in the lower zones, in contrast to smoking-related emphysema, but it can affect all lung fields. Only a minority of homozygous A1AD develop severe liver disease, but some patients may present with neonatal jaundice. Other organ manifestations of A1AD include relapsing panniculitis, vasculitis and glomerulonephritis. Treatment of A1AD is similar to standard COPD therapy with smoking cessation particularly emphasized. α1-Antitrypsin is not routinely replaced. Lung and/or liver transplant may be options for some patients. A1AD patients should be managed at a specialist centre and their family should be offered genetic counselling.

KEY POINTS

- Acute exacerbation of COPD is a common acute medical emergency that should be recognized and treated promptly.
- α1-Antitrypsin deficiency is one of the most commonly inherited genetic disorders. Smoking cessation is the key in halting its lung manifestations.

CASE 67: COFFEE-GROUND VOMITING

History
A 78-year-old man has been admitted with a one-day history of coffee-ground vomiting and black, tarry stools. His medical history is significant for hypertension and osteo-arthritis. He regularly takes diclofenac 50 mg three times a day to control his knee pain, as well as aspirin 75 mg and bendroflumethiazide 2.5 mg once daily.

Examination
This man felt cool up to the wrists and his pulse volume was reduced. His jugular venous pulse (JVP) was not visible. Respiratory and abdominal examinations were unremarkable. Per rectal examination confirmed fresh melaena. The patient's haemoglobin level on admission was 8.2 g/dL (normal range 13–17 g/dL).

Initial treatment
An oesophagoduodenoscopy (OGD) was performed and showed a large duodenal ulcer with surrounding areas of bleeding. It was injected with adrenaline. He has been treated with intravenous proton pump inhibitors to aid ulcer healing. Twelve hours after his OGD he was found to have further melaena. He is feeling unwell and dizzy. Observations at this time: temperature 37.2°C, heart rate 128/min irregular, blood pressure 100/65 mmHg, respiratory rate 24/min, SaO_2 98 per cent on room air, Glasgow Coma Scale score 15/15.

INVESTIGATIONS		
		Normal range
On admission (repeat samples awaited)		
White cells	7.2	$4–11 \times 10^9$/L
Haemoglobin	8.0	13–18 g/dL
Platelets	450	$150–400 \times 10^9$/L
Sodium	130	135–145 mmol/L
Potassium	3.2	3.5–5.0 mmol/L
Urea	24.0	3.0–7.0 mmol/L
Creatinine	180	60–110 µmol/L
C-reactive protein	10	<5 mg/L
Alanine aminotransferase	56	8–55 IU/L
Alkaline phosphatase	100	42–98 IU/L
INR	1.2	0.9–1.1
Arterial blood gas on room air:		
pH	7.35	7.35–7.45
PO_2	12.2	9.3–13.3 kPa
PCO_2	3.9	4.7–6.0 kPa
Lactate	3	<2 mmol/L
HCO_3	3	22–26 mmol/L
Base excess	−4	−3 to +3 mmol/L
Haemoglobin	6.2	13–18 g/dL

Question
- What would be the appropriate management of this patient?

This man has had a further episode of melaena and, on examination, he is cool to the touch and shows signs of depleted fluid volume (reduced pulse volume and low JVP). The arterial blood gas sample shows an elevated lactate, an even lower haemoglobin and a borderline metabolic acidosis, all of which are highly suggestive of re-bleeding of the duodenal ulcer found on the OGD. The first management step is to resuscitate his hypo-volaemic state and correct any clotting disorder that may contribute to his bleeding. The second step should include bleeding source control through repeat OGD.

The symptoms and signs are highly suggestive of hypovolaemia. It is important to support the circulation with intravenous fluid, so first ensure that multiple good intravenous accesses are available. The best intravenous fluid in this situation is red cell transfusion, so emergency cross-matching should be requested. In critical situations 'crash blood' can be used and is usually available in the accident and emergency department, labour ward or the blood bank. In the interim, crystalloid and colloid solutions should be used to resuscitate the circulation. Bolus colloid challenge is preferable when blood pressure is unstable. Where facilities allow, an arterial line should be inserted to allow continuous blood pressure monitoring. The target mean arterial pressure for resuscitation should not be excessively high to avoid exacerbating bleeding. Central venous access performed under ultrasound guidance should be considered in patients with other co-morbidity such as renal failure or congestive cardiac failure, although it is not the intravenous access of choice in urgent resuscitation as it takes time to insert and drip rate is lower than large bore peripheral venous catheter. A urinary catheter should be inserted to monitor urine output and as a crude assessment of organ perfusion.

Since his pulse is irregular, a 12-lead ECG should be performed to look for arrhythmia such as atrial fibrillation. New atrial fibrillation in a critically unwell patient usually responds to treatment of the underlying cause – in this case hypovolaemia. Antiarrhythmic treatment should only be considered if the arrhythmia is impairing organ perfusion despite adequate fluid resuscitation. Amiodarone or digoxin should be used as they have relatively mild or no negative inotropic effects.

In acute bleeding the target haemoglobin for transfusion is often set higher (e.g. 9 g/dL). The clotting cascade should be optimized with products such as platelets, fresh frozen plasma and cryoprecipitate to ensure platelets $>50 \times 10^9$/L, INR <1.4, and fibrinogen >1.4 g/L. Liaison with the haematology team is often helpful in these situations. The use of tranexamic acid has increased since the publication of the CRASH-2 trial which found a positive outcome with the use of tranexamic acid in trauma patients. Tranexamic acid is a potent fibrinolytic inhibitor which is cost-effective, but its efficacy has not been proven in the setting of upper gastrointestinal bleeding.

The optimal timing of proton pump inhibitor therapy initiation is currently not known with patients presenting with non-variceal bleeding. However, it is clear that, once a peptic ulcer is confirmed, high-dose intravenous proton pump inhibitor (initial loading dose with continuous infusion for 72 hours) should be prescribed as soon as possible.

The Rockall score is a validated system designed to predict mortality from upper gastrointestinal bleeding. As per the national guideline, it should be calculated pre-endoscopy to assess risk and decide urgency of endoscopy. A pre-endoscopic Rockall score greater than 3 is deemed significant. In this case, calculating Rockall score for re-bleeding is probably unnecessary as re-bleeding itself is already a good indication of significant risk of mortality and it should be dealt with urgently.

While ongoing resuscitation takes place, the on-call endoscopist and surgeons should be contacted. Surgery may have a role in gastrointestinal bleeding when it is not controlled by endoscopy alone.

Helicobacter pylori is associated with 80–95 per cent of duodenal ulcers without a history of non-steroidal anti-inflammatory drug use. Its prevalence is lower in patients with duodenal ulcers related to NSAIDs. In the acute phase, empirical antibiotics are probably unnecessary as they do not reduce the immediate bleeding risk. A CLO (Campylobacter-like organism) test is often carried out to detect *H. pylori* infection. Once tested positive, a triple therapy consisting of two antibiotics and an ulcer healing agent should be started to reduce the future risk of ulcer reformation. Repeat OGD is often carried out with high-risk bleeding or re-bleeding. However, in stable patients repeat OGD is necessary only with gastric ulcers to look for evidence of underlying malignancy.

 KEY POINTS

- Re-bleeding in the context of gastrointestinal bleeding carries significant mortality.
- Prompt circulatory resuscitation and source control (endoscopy or surgery) should be carried out as soon as feasible.

History

A 32-year-old man was admitted to a psychiatric ward one week earlier for inpatient treatment of acute psychosis. He was managed with haloperidol 5 mg intramuscularly every 8 hours and lorazepam 1 mg p.r.n for sedation. He had been progressing well up until yesterday, when he complained of progressive dysphagia and muscle stiffness. Over the course of the day he developed a temperature (38.5°C) and has became increasingly drowsy.

Examination

This patient is unkempt and drowsy. Cardiovascular, respiratory and abdominal examinations are unremarkable. His Glasgow Coma Scale score is 11/15 (E3, V3, M5). Cranial nerve examination is difficult to perform, but no obvious abnormality is detected. The peripheral nervous system examination is significant for increased tone. Reflexes are difficult to elicit. He has had a low urine output. Observations: heart rate 132/min, blood pressure 140/85 mmHg.

INVESTIGATIONS		
		Normal range
White cells	16.0	$4–11 \times 10^9$/L
Haemoglobin	15.0	13–18 g/dL
Platelets	184	$150–400 \times 10^9$/L
Sodium	135	135–145 mmol/L
Potassium	7.0	3.5–5.0 mmol/L
Urea	20	3.0–7.0 mmol/L
Creatinine	300	60–110 µmol/L
C-reactive protein	12	<5 mg/L
INR	1.8	0.9–1.1
Lactate dehydrogenase	1258	50–150 IU
Creatine kinase	9988	38–300 IU
Corrected Ca^{2+}	1.9	2.2–2.65 mmol/L
Arterial blood gas on room air:		
pH	7.26	7.35–7.45
PO_2	14.0	9.3–13.3 kPa
PCO_2	3.5	4.7–6.0 kPa
Lactate	2.3	<2 mmol/L
HCO_3	15	22–26 mmol/L
Base excess	−9	−3 to +3 mmol/L
Urine dipstick:	Blood 4+, protein 1+	

Questions
- What is the most likely diagnosis?
- How would you manage this patient?

ANSWER 68

This man has findings highly suggestive of neuroleptic malignant syndrome (NMS). The main differential diagnoses include malignant hyperthermia and serotonin syndrome, but the temporal relationship of antipsychotics makes this diagnosis more likely. NMS normally presents 1–3 days after initiation of antipsychotics but patients remain at risk of NMS for at least 10–20 days, even if antipsychotics are stopped. NMS is a medical emergency and this patient's biochemistry is highly suggestive of a secondary acute kidney injury and rhabdomyolysis. The hyperkalaemia is particularly worrying, as this puts him at risk of cardiac arrhythmias.

Only a small subset of patients are at risk of NMS. Dopamine is central to thermoregulation and muscle tone. Blocking central dopaminergic receptors in these patients can cause deranged temperature control and abnormal calcium handling. There is also direct toxicity to the muscle fibres, which leads to hyperthermia and muscle rigidity. The creatine kinase (CK) and lactate dehydrogenase (LDH) have become elevated due to muscle necrosis and cell breakdown. Rhabdomyolysis (the breaking down of muscle fibres) leads to the release of myoglobin and other products into the bloodstream and these often precipitate an acute kidney injury.

The diagnostic criteria of NMS are as follows (require 3 major OR 2 major and 4 minor):

- major – fever, muscle rigidity, elevated CK;
- minor – abnormal blood pressure, tachycardia, tachypnoea, altered consciousness, leucocytosis, diaphoresis.

The finding of haematuria on urine dipstick is likely to be due to myoglobinuria rather than true haematuria. However, only 50 per cent of patients present with myoglobinuria. Increased purine metabolism and subsequent hepatic conversion causes hyperuricaemia. Potassium and phosphate released from muscle necrosis and the subsequent hyperphosphataemia chelate serum calcium, leading to hypocalcaemia. Treatment of hyperkalaemia should be urgent, but abnormal urate and calcium and phosphate levels are usually managed conservatively. It is also important to check the patient's INR, D-dimer level, fibrinogen level and platelet count to look for evidence of disseminated intravascular coagulation (DIC), a known complication of severe rhabdomyolysis.

In this patient, the key priorities of his mangement should be (i) stopping the offending drugs and all other unnecessary medications that may worsen hyperkalaemia and renal function (beta-blockers and digoxin should be withheld as they reduce the efficacy of insulin treatment and intracellular potassium buffering); (ii) aggressive fluid resuscitation; (iii) management of hyperkalaemia; and (iv) temperature control. He should be managed in a high-dependency area with airway monitoring as he appeared drowsy on presentation. Full non-invasive cardiorespiratory monitoring is crucial to look for evidence of malignant arrhythmias secondary to hyperkalaemia. Intravenous access should be secured and crystalloid fluid (e.g. 0.9% saline) should be given as a fluid challenge (i.e. 1 L over 30–60 minutes). A 12-lead ECG should be obtained immediately. Without delay, 10 mL of 10% calcium gluconate (or calcium chloride, whichever is accessible) should be given over 2–5 minutes, and 10 units of insulin with 20% glucose in 100 mL should be given over 5–15 minutes (extravasation of 50% glucose into tissues is highly toxic, so 20% glucose in a larger volume is preferable). Calcium gluconate should be repeated every 10 minutes until hyperkalaemic ECG changes are resolved. The effect of insulin/glucose should occur in 15 minutes and last for 4 hours. The maximum reduction of potassium is 1.0 mmol/L. Glucose should be monitored regularly as hypoglycaemia could potentially be a problem up to 6 hours after insulin treatment.

Other useful medications for hyperkalaemia are salbutamol 10 mg in divided doses via nebulizers (over 30 minutes or 1 hour). Note that salbutamol may precipitate myocardial ischaemia. It has the potential to reduce potassium by 1.0 mmol/L and its effects last up to 2 hours. Response to salbutamol is less reliable compared with calcium gluconate and insulin/glucose. The potassium should be re-checked after treatment. Urgent renal replacement therapy should be considered for metabolic acidosis, refractory hyperkalaemia and anuria despite fluid resuscitation.

The key to management of rhabdomyolysis is large-volume crystalloid fluid resuscitation. Up to 6–10 L/day may be required for 3–5 days. Fluid overload can be treated by furosemide. If anuria develops, urgent renal replacement should be considered.

Other treatment for NMS entails core temperature reduction using cooling blankets and antipyretics. The value of other interventions, such as dantrolene and bromocriptine, remains uncertain, although dantroline may be useful in patients with refractory hyperthermia.

Managing this patient's psychosis may be difficult and close liaison with the psychiatry team may be necessary.

 KEY POINTS

- Neuroleptic malignant sydrome usually presents within a week of commencing antipsychotic medication.
- Symptoms include pyrexia and rigidity, and management with fluids and cooling therapies should be commenced as soon as the diagnosis is made.

CASE 69: RESPIRATORY DISTRESS AND OEDEMA

History

A 78-year-old woman has presented to the emergency department with acute severe shortness of breath and wheeze. Over the past 2 hours this has been increasingly severe. She has no chest pain, cough or fever. Her medical history includes hypertension, peripheral vascular disease and chronic kidney disease stage 4. Over the past year her estimated glomerular filtration rate has deteriorated by two-thirds and her hypertension has become more treatment-resistant, accompanied by reduced exercise tolerance, orthopnoea and bilateral lower limb oedema. Of note, this is her third similar presentation to the hospital in the past year. She is taking several drugs: hydralazine, 50 mg thrice daily; isosorbide mononitrate, 60 mg once daily; nebivolol, 5 mg once daily; spironolactone, 25 mg once daily; furosemide, 80 mg twice daily; amlodipine, 10 mg once daily; aspirin, 75 mg once daily; atorvastatin, 10 mg once daily. She has no known drug allergies.

Examination

This elderly woman is in respiratory distress and immediate high-flow oxygen is provided. There is peripheral oedema up to her knees. Her pulse is regular, jugular venous pressure (JVP) raised at 11 cm. On auscultation her heart sounds are normal. There are inspiratory crackles up to the mid-zone bilaterally and mild end-expiratory wheeze. An ECG shows left ventricular hypertrophy with straining. Echocardiography shows concentric left ventricular hypertrophy (E/A ratio 0.5, ejection fraction 55 per cent; no valvular abnormality). A chest X-ray is

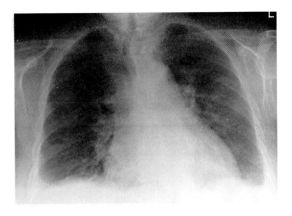

Figure 69.1

shown in Fig. 69.1. Observations: temperature 37°C, heart rate 86/min, blood pressure 180/110 mmHg, respiratory rate 38/min, SaO_2 91 per cent on room air.

INVESTIGATIONS		
		Normal range
Sodium	134	135–145 mmol/L
Potassium	5.0	3.5–5.0 mmol/L
Urea	22.6	3.0–7.0 mmol/L
Creatinine	300	60–110 µmol/L
C-reactive protein	<5	<5 mg/L
Urine dipstick:		
Protein 3+		
Blood: nitrite negative, leucocyte negative, no protein		

Questions
• What is the differential diagnosis?
• What is the appropriate management?

ANSWER 69

The differential diagnoses of acute shortness of breath and wheeze include acute exacerbation of obstructive airway diseases and acute pulmonary oedema. In this case the history, examination and chest radiograph findings are consistent with acute pulmonary oedema. Note the upper-lobe blood diversion and the fluffy infiltrates throughout the lung fields suggestive of pulmonary oedema, as well as the blunted costophrenic angles, indicating small pleural effusions, which are probably due to fluid overload.

The treatments of acute pulmonary oedema include high-flow oxygen and intravenous morphine or diamorphine to relieve the drowning sensation associated with pulmonary oedema. In addition, morphine has a modest venodilating effect. Intravenous furosemide and glyceryl trinitrate are the mainstay to relieve fluid retention and allow a balanced vasodilation, respectively, to aid the failing heart. Non-invasive continuous positive airway pressure (CPAP) ventilation can be used and is shown to be beneficial in the treatment of acute pulmonary oedema. It is always important to look for the underlying causes of acute pulmonary oedema such as acute coronary syndrome or arrhythmia. Once over the acute phase, a transthoracic echocardiogram will be a useful tool to look for valvular heart diseases, structural defect of the myocardium and ventricular performance.

Her recent history of resistant hypertension, worsening renal impairment, fluid retention, proteinuria and recurrent presentation of pulmonary oedema are collectively pointing towards renovascular disease as the underlying aetiology of her recent deterioration. 'Flash pulmonary oedema' is a term used to describe circulatory overload out of proportion to left ventricular systolic function and is often ascribed to underlying haemodynamically significant renal artery stenosis (RAS).

It is important to note the conceptual difference between the condition RAS and renovascular disease (RVD). Renal artery stenosis is often found on angiography incidentally when patients undergo angiography for another reason, and not all lesions (especially those with <50 per cent lumen occlusion) cause RVD. True RVD is defined by the elevation of blood pressure in the presence of haemodynamically significant RAS. Most RVD cases are managed medically with antihypertensive medications, and not all RAS needs surgical or radiological intervention. In fact the treatment of RAS remains a topic of debate as not all patients undergoing interventions for RAS will have better control of blood pressure or recovery of renal function.

RAS is commonly caused by atherosclerotic lesions or fibromuscular dysplasia in the large renal arteries and its branches. Frequently diffuse atherosclerosis also affects smaller vessels which are not detectable on radiological or angiographic studies. Fibromuscular dysplasia can affect any age group but it is found more commonly in young females. Owing to the autoregulatory mechanisms of renal vascular beds, the degree of stenosis does not correlate well with reduction in glomerular filtration rate (GFR); hence the difficulty in deciding how much an impact a stenotic lesion has on the kidneys.

One of the main effects of renovascular disease is resistant hypertension and this is driven by activation of the renin–angiotensin–aldosterone system (RAA) and reduction in pressure natriuresis. In renovascular disease, renin is often elevated as a result of ischaemia from reduction in blood flow. This leads to activation of the RAA cascade. The increase in circulating angiotensin II has a direct effect of increased vasoconstriction and also activation of aldosterone, which leads to salt and water retention. This increase in blood pressure helps the kidney to restore pressure natriuresis, but with time this compensatory mechanism also begins to fail and the reduction in flow beyond the stenotic lesion becomes significant and there is a reduction in pressure natriuresis, leading to further salt and water retention.

The main goals of treatments for RVD are similar to those of other vascular disease: risk factor reduction such as smoking cessation, blood pressure and cholesterol control and other lifestyle modifications. A combination of antihypertensives is often needed to adequately control blood pressure. Angiotensin-converting enzyme (ACE) inhibitors or angiotensin receptor blockers (ARBs) should be used with caution as stenotic lesions (especially in bilateral RAS) may be highly dependent on circulating angiotensin II to maintain glomerular filtration. ACEs/ARBs have higher efficacy in dilating efferent arterioles than afferent arterioles in the glomeruli, resulting in reduction in glomerular filtration and worsening renal impairment. ACEs/ARBs should be withheld if their introduction leads to hyperkalaemia or more than 20 per cent rise in creatinine.

In deciding whether a patient will benefit from radiological or surgical intervention, it is important to assess the haemodynamic significance of RAS and whether there will be reasonable chance to improve renal function. Captopril renography and CT renal angiography are common non-invasive investigations, but conventional angiography remains the gold standard for evaluation of RAS. Note that angiography in general uses contrast that may precipitate acute kidney injury, so the risk benefit is often discussed prior to proceeding with this procedure.

 KEY POINTS

- Acute pulmonary oedema is a common medical emergency that should be promptly recognized and treated.
- The definitive treatment of renovascular disease remains controversial. Control of reversible cardiovascular risk such as smoking cessation, cholesterol and blood pressure lowering may slow down the progression of renovascular disease.

History

A 35-year-old man has presented with a severe burn to his right hand. He tipped some boiling water on to the hand a few hours earlier, which led to severe erythema and blisters, but he does not complain of any pain from the injury. Over the last month he has experienced mild shoulder pain, exacerbated by coughing, and bilateral leg stiffness resulting in walking difficulty. He works as a librarian. He has no medical, drug, travel or smoking histories. He drinks fewer than 10 units of alcohol per week.

Examination

Cardiorespiratory and abdominal examinations are unremarkable. There is no rash or lymphadenopathy. Cranial nerve examination is normal, and no spinal tenderness is elicited. In the upper limb, tone is normal. His hands appear to have slight wasting bilaterally, with mild weakness, but other myotomes are within normal limits. There is no wrist tenderness. Reflexes in the arms are absent. Light touch sensation is intact throughout the upper limbs, but pain sensation is absent bilaterally from C4 to T4 distribution. In the lower limbs, the tone is elevated with ankle clonus bilaterally. Power is globally reduced to 4/5 (Medical Research Council scale), and there is hyper-reflexia. All sensation modalities are intact in the lower limbs. Coordination and vibration sense are preserved in all limbs. Anal tone and perineal sensation are intact. A chest X-ray shows no abnormalities. Observations: temperature 36.5°C, heart rate 80/min, blood pressure 105/70 mmHg, SaO_2 100 per cent on room air.

INVESTIGATIONS		
		Normal range
White cells	6.0	$4–11 \times 10^9$/L
Neutrophils	2.8	$2–7 \times 10^9$/L
Haemoglobin	13.0	13–18 g/dL
Platelets	250	$150–400 \times 10^9$/L
Sodium	137	135–145 mmol/L
Potassium	4.5	3.5–5.0 mmol/L
Urea	4.6	3.0–7.0 mmol/L
Creatinine	73	60–110 µmol/L
C-reactive protein	300	<5 mg/L
Bilirubin	20	5–25 µmol/L
Alanine transaminase	35	8–55 IU/L
Alkaline phosphatase	180	42–98 IU/L
Albumin	35	35–50 g/L
Creatine kinase	88	60–320 IU/L
Erythrocyte sedimentation rate	<10	Males, age/2; females, [age+10]/2
Antinuclear antibodies	Negative	
Antinuclear cytoplasmic antibodies	Negative	

Questions

- What is the differential diagnosis?
- What should be the management plan?

In approaching a neurological case, it is important to try to localize where the lesion(s) are within the neurological system. When investigating weakness it can be divided into:

- myopathy (i.e. not a neurological disorder);
- neuromuscular junction disorder;
- peripheral nerve;
- radiculopathy/spinal cord lesion/myelopathy;
- lesion in the brainstem and/or cerebellum;
- cortical lesion.

The patterns of presentation differ and this helps to localize the lesion.

This patient's neurological findings can be summarized as:

- spastic paraparesis in the lower limbs (as demonstrated by bilateral upper motor neuron signs);
- dissociated sensory loss in the upper limbs (i.e. spinothalamic impairment but intact posterior column);
- absent upper-limb reflexes with hand-muscle wasting.

Putting all this together suggests the lesion is within the spinal cord at the level of the cervical and upper thoracic cord. This will produce a segmental effect, as demonstrated by lower motor neuron signs in the upper limbs and long-tract effect, as demonstrated by upper motor neuron signs below the level of the spinal cord lesion.

Having established the site of lesion within the neurological system, the next step is to find out what type of cord lesion this is. The common causes of cord lesions are tumours, infection, disc disease and spondylosis, haematoma or cystic lesions. Except for disc disease and spondylosis, most of these pathological processes can occur in the extradural, intradural or intramedullary space. All lesions within the spinal cord can produce local segmental damage and long-tract effects (i.e. damage/interruption to ascending and descending tracts within the cord).

With regard to local segmental damage, the lesions can affect (i) a nerve root (radiculopathy), which leads to severe, sharp, shooting, burning pain at that nerve root distribution and is aggravated by movement, straining and coughing; or (ii) cord (myelopathy), leading to dull ache which is continuous, unaffected by movement and may radiate into the whole leg or even one half of the body. Bone pathology tends to cause localized tenderness which is reproducible by palpation of the affected area. For long-tract effects, the effects are dependent on which long tract is affected (spinothalamic, posterior column, spinocerebellar or corticospinal tracts). In addition, damage to the sympathetic outflow at level of T1 or the cervical cord may lead to Horner's syndrome. Bladder symptoms occur when both sides of the spinal cord are affected; usually they start with difficulty in initiating micturition before retention symptoms develop.

The combinations of presenting symptoms are also reflective of segmental damage within the affected cord. Cord lesion can be divided into (i) extrinsic compressive lesions, (ii) central cord lesions, (iii) cauda equina lesions. For extrinsic compressive lesions, the long-tract effects depend on the location of the tumour. For example, a posterior tumour causes ipsilateral posterior column lesions first (light touch, proprioception and vibration sensory loss) and, as it expands, it may cause further direct pressure effects or ischaemia to the neighbouring tracts – so it may cause ipsilateral corticospinal tract lesions (upper motor neuron signs) and then contralateral spinothalamic tract lesions (pain and temperature loss). If half of the spinal cord is affected then it produces a combination of symptoms consistent with Brown–Séquard syndrome.

In contrast with extrinsic compressive lesions, the central cord lesions produce a different set of long-tract signs. The centrality of the lesion means that the medially situated fibres are involved first. As the spinothalamic tract decussates at the level of the spinal cord, central cord lesions cause bilateral sensory loss at the level of the lesion initially. With a cervical central cord lesion the pattern of spinothalamic damage may expand to a 'cape' or 'suspended' pattern (with pain and temperature sensory deficit spared in the sacral distribution even with large central lesion) due to the peripheral location of sacral fibres within the spinothalamic tract. As the central cord lesion expands, corticospinal tracts are involved leading to lower motor neuron lesions at the level of spinal cord affected (e.g. hand-muscle wasting) and upper motor neuron signs below the level of lesions (e.g. spastic paraparesis). Posterior column signs appear late.

Cauda equina lesions typically affect the lumbosacral areas. If lesions are affecting the sacral nerve roots they cause saddle anaesthesia and bladder symptoms earlier than other lesions.

This man's symptoms and signs are consistent with a central spinal cord lesion. The combination of dissociated sensory loss and spastic paraparesis is highly suggestive of a cystic lesion known as syringomyelia. Other differential diagnoses are cystic intramedullary tumours, infection and haematoma. Subacute combined degeneration of the cord and multiple sclerosis can sometimes produce a similar collection of symptoms.

Syringomyelia is a rare disorder with a prevalence of 8.4 cases per 100 000 population. An abnormal cerebrospinal fluid-filled cavity known as a syrinx develops in the spinal cord. If a syrinx develops within the brainstem, the condition is termed syringobulbia. Syringomyelia is associated with Arnold–Chiari malformation which is a developmental abnormality of the brainstem and cerebellum: the cerebellar tonsils herniate through the foramen magnum. The pathophysiology of syringomyelia is incompletely understood.

Magnetic resonance imaging of the brain and spinal cord is the investigation of choice (Fig. 70.1), which will demonstrate the characteristic syrinx, the extent of the lesion and rule out other conditions as mentioned above. Cerebrospinal fluid (CSF) sampling is relatively contraindicated owing to the risk of herniation. The natural history of this condition is variable and neurosurgery is considered but is not curative because, despite best effort, at least 33 per cent of patients suffer progressive deterioration.

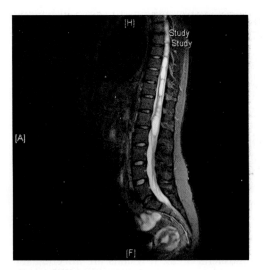

Figure 70.1

History

A 65-year-old man has presented to the emergency department with a one-day history of generalized headache, shortness of breath, fever, rigors, productive cough, right-sided pleuritic chest pain, myalgia and watery diarrhoea. He returned from Kuala Lumpur three days ago after a five-day holiday with his family. He stayed in the city and did not visit the countryside. His hotel was air-conditioned and he ate cooked meals there. His wife, who was travelling with him, also presented with a similar illness. He is normally fit and well with no past medical history.

Examination

The man is visibly tachypnoeic and appears disorientated in time and place. There is no rash nor signs of meningeal irritation. He feels hot to the touch and his pulse is fast and regular but bounding in character. On auscultation of his chest there is bronchial breathing and coarse crackles in the right mid and lower zones posteriorly. The rest of the cardiorespiratory, abdominal and neurological examinations are unremarkable. A chest X-ray is shown in Fig. 71.1.Observations: temperature 40°C, heart rate 130/min, blood pressure 108/55 mmHg, respiratory rate 32/min, SaO_2 90 per cent on room air.

INVESTIGATIONS		
		Normal range
White cells	20.0	$4–11 \times 10^9$/L
Neutrophils	18	$2–7 \times 10^9$/L
Haemoglobin	15.0	13–18 g/dL
Platelets	188	$150–400 \times 10^9$/L
Sodium	129	135–145 mmol/L
Potassium	3.9	3.5–5.0 mmol/L
Urea	15	3.0–7.0 mmol/L
Creatinine	155	60–110 µmol/L
C-reactive protein	300	<5 mg/L
Bilirubin	20	5–25 µmol/L
Alanine aminotransferase	35	8–55 IU/L
Alkaline phosphatase	180	42–98 IU/L
Albumin	35	35–50 g/L
Creatine kinase	568	60–320 IU/L
Arterial blood gas on air:		
pH	7.48	7.35–7.45
PO_2	7.9	9.3–13.3 kPa
PCO_2	3.2	4.7–6.0 kPa
Lactate	4.0	<2 mmol/L
HCO_3	24	22–26 mmol/L
Base excess	−3	−3 to +3 mmol/L

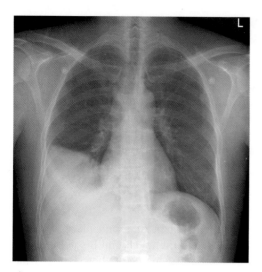

Figure 71.1

Questions

- What is the diagnosis?
- What should be the management plan?

This man's clinical presentation and investigation results are highly suggestive of community-acquired pneumonia. He has bronchial breathing indicating consolidation. His chest X-ray shows opacification in the right lower zone. This obscures the diaphragm but not the right heart border, indicating that it is likely to be in the right lower lobe. It contains an air bronchogram confirming consolidation.

CURB 65 is one of the most commonly used tools for assessment of community-acquired pneumonia severity. It is a useful adjunct but should not replace thorough clinical assessment. CURB 65 stands for: C = confusion; U = Urea ≥7 mmol/L; R = Respiratory rate >30/min; B = Blood pressure systolic <90 or diastolic <60 mmHg; 65 = age ≥65 years. Mortality approaches 83 per cent if all four CURB components are present. CURB 65 is also a useful tool to decide whether to manage a patient with pneumonia in the community or in a hospital environment. When the patient is managed in the community, appropriate patient and/or relative education and clinical review mechanisms should be in place.

The most important initial management plan is to ensure his hypoxia is corrected by high-flow oxygen as swiftly as possible. Intravenous fluids should also be prescribed. He should be monitored in a high-dependency area with continuous cardiorespiratory and urine output monitoring. The aim is to ensure oxygen saturation is >94 per cent and respiratory rate <30/min. It is also important to monitor for clinical signs of respiratory depression secondary to exhaustion. Patients with persistent hypoxia, signs of exhaustion or shock should be transferred to a critical-care unit as soon as possible for intubation and intermittent positive pressure ventilation and circulatory support. In respiratory failure secondary to pneumonia, non-invasive mask/helmet continuous positive airway pressure devices are a useful adjunct while awaiting invasive ventilation, but this should not delay intubation.

Antibiotics should be given at the earliest opportunity and should be no later than 4 hours after presentation to hospital. As with all antibiotic prescriptions, it is essential to establish history of antibiotic allergy. When taking an allergy history it is important to establish the nature of the drug allergy. If the allergy history is unclear it is important to avoid the class of drugs in the acute setting with a view to allergy testing to clarify the nature of the allergy when the patient has recovered. Microbiology investigations including sputum and blood cultures should be taken, although it should not delay the initiation of antibiotics. Performing sputum cultures whilst on antibiotic treatment is unlikely to be helpful. In all severe cases of pneumonia, urinary pneumococcal antigen, urinary *Legionella* antigen and *Mycoplasma* sputum polymerase chain reaction (PCR) assay should be considered. Pleuritic chest pain and fever should be managed by paracetamol or other simple analgesics.

This man has presented with classic symptoms of fever with evidence of extrapulmonary manifestations such as headache, myalgia and watery diarrhoea. His blood test also reveals an elevated liver enzyme profile and acute kidney injury. While all these features could be consistent with severe pneumonia leading to multi-organ injury or failure, atypical pneumonia should be suspected. Atypical pneumonia is not a distinctive clinical syndrome. Most if not all atypical pneumonias present with classical pneumonic symptoms (fever, productive cough and shortness of breath), so it is hard to differentiate clinically. Atypical pneumonia is a term used to describe pneumonia caused by (i) *Mycoplasma pneumoniae*, (ii) *Chlamydophila pneumoniae*, (iii) *Chlamydophila psittaci*,

(iv) *Coxiella burnetii*, (v) *Legionella* spp, or (vi) *Francisella tularensi*. The term 'atypical pneumonia' remains useful to describe these pathogens as their treatment and sometimes duration of antibiotic therapy is different from typical pathogens. Atypical pathogens are intracellular pathogens and lack a bacterial cell wall, so they are not susceptible to β-lactam-based antibiotics. Atypical pneumonias are normally treated with macrolides, quinolones or tetracycline classes of antibiotics.

In this case it is reasonable to suspect Legionnaire's disease from the travel history and a similar illness suffered by his wife. *Legionella* spp are a group of Gram-negative rods that are obligate or facultative intracellular bacteria. Transmission is usually via contaminated aerosol inhalation. Around half the cases are travel-related, and most UK cases occur predominantly over August and October each year from a combination of environmental and human behaviour over summer months. *Legionella* spp thrive in the warmer waters of summer, and over this period there is usually an increased use of cooling towers and air-conditioning units so that transmission is more frequent. *Legionella* infection has two distinctive clinical patterns. It can cause a rapid progressive illness and is seen more frequently in critically ill patients. It can also cause a mild self-limiting illness termed 'Pontiac fever'. The more severe form of *Legionella* disease can often lead to gastrointestinal, cardiac and central nervous system manifestations, although other atypical organisms such as *Chlamydophila psittaci*, *Coxiella burnetii* and *Mycoplasma pneumoniae* have distinctive extrapulmonary manifestations too.

In all patients diagnosed with community-acquired pneumonia, follow-up chest radiograph six weeks after the initial illness should be considered if there are persisting symptoms or clinical signs or a high risk of underlying malignancy. It is also important to note that *Legionella* is a notifiable illness and all cases should be reported as per Health Protection Agency policy.

 KEY POINTS

- *Legionella* disease is a notifiable illness.
- It should be suspected in cases of severe community-acquired pneumonia.

History

An 82-year-old woman had noticed increasing difficulty over recent months when trying to go up stairs. She was awaiting a hip replacement and suffered from hip pain, which she managed with paracetamol and codeine. One evening she tripped and fell down eight stairs, sustaining a large laceration to the scalp which bled profusely. She called her daughter who phoned for an ambulance. On arrival at hospital she was alert and orientated and appeared well. A systems examination was unremarkable.

Initial treatment

Her laceration was stitched and she was keen to go home. She was assessed by the physiotherapy and occupational therapy teams who felt it would be safer to keep her as an inpatient until aids to manage the stairs had been fitted.

Examination

This woman was mobilizing around the ward and was independent with self-care, but three days later she was found to be confused and drowsy in bed. Her symptoms progressed, and within 4 hours her pupils were only sluggishly responding to light and she was unrousable. Her heart rate had fallen from 88 to 40/min and her blood pressure had risen from 110/60 to 183/75 mmHg. Her respiratory rate had increased from 15 to 26 breaths per minute, and her oxygen requirements increased until her saturations were 91 per cent on 15 L oxygen. She was assessed by the junior elderly-care doctor on-call who arranged an urgent CT head scan (Fig. 72.1). Her observation chart is shown in Fig. 72.2.

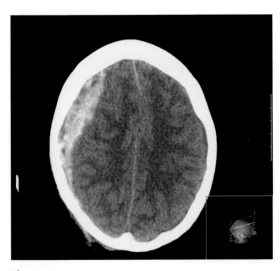

Figure 72.1

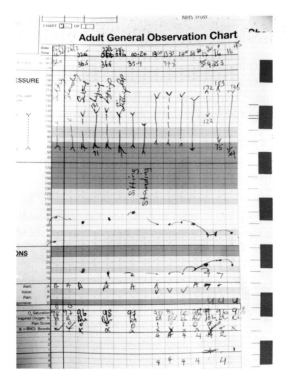

Figure 72.2

Questions

- What would you suspect with symptoms like this?
- What treatment can be given to a patient with these problems?

ANSWER 72

The main differential diagnosis is a chronic subdural haematoma. Subdural haematomas are bleeds that occur between the dura mater and the arachnoid mater, enveloping the brain. They usually develop following traumatic injury, as with this case. The bridging veins crossing the subdural space tear when head injuries take place, mainly due to the high-speed accelerations and decelerations that occur. Older people are particularly prone to such injuries as the brain naturally atrophies and shrinks with age. Blood collects in the space and draws in water due to osmotic pressures. The area of bleeding increases in size, causing compression of the cerebral tissue.

This patient has signs of raised intracranial pressure, as noted by the change in her bedside observations (see Fig. 72.2). Cushing's triad of systolic hypertension with a wide pulse pressure, bradycardia and irregular or rapid respiratory rate is a major sign of raised intracranial pressure. These features occur due to insufficient blood flow to the brain and compression of arterioles.

Subacute and chronic subdural haematomas classically present days to weeks after the insult. Any patient who presents with neurological signs several days after a head injury should be investigated for a subdural bleed.

Ideally, bleeds should be identified as soon as possible. Any patient with a head injury should undergo a neurological examination and, if abnormal signs are present, a CT head scan should be considered. Small bleeds may be monitored over time, as if the bleeding has stopped, neurosurgical intervention may not be required. Larger bleeds may require a hole to be drilled into the skull to remove a blood clot, or a craniotomy can be performed. Unfortunately, as in this advanced case of a bleed, the haematoma may be inoperable and palliative care will be commenced.

 KEY POINTS

- Always perform a full neurological examination of anyone presenting with a head injury.
- Have a low threshold for considering a subdural bleed in patients who deteriorate more than 48 hours after their head injury.

History

A 64-year-old woman was admitted to hospital with shortness of breath and a cough productive of dark green sputum. She was treated in the emergency department with intravenous fluid rehydration and a penicillin-based antibiotic. Five minutes after administration of the antibiotic she complained of feeling short of breath and dizzy. She sounded wheezy and looked very pale. An erythematous, macular rash is noted on her face and trunk.

Examination

Nurse observations: temperature 37.5°C, heart rate 130/min, blood pressure 80/42 mmHg, respiratory rate 24/min, SaO_2 96 per cent on room air.

Questions

- What is the most likely diagnosis?
- How would you manage this patient acutely?
- Once she is stabilized, what management plan would you suggest?

This woman is likely to be having an anaphylactic reaction to the penicillin-based antibiotic. Anaphylaxis is a systemic reaction to an allergen, leading to degranulation of mast cells and basophils and the release of histamine and other inflammatory mediators. Initial clinical features can include rash, facial swelling, hypotension, tachycardia and wheeze, which can progress to laryngeal oedema, bronchospasm and circulatory collapse. This is a life-threatening condition and needs to be recognized and treated urgently.

The acute management of anaphylaxis can be life-saving and should be commenced as soon as you suspect the diagnosis. In a hospital-based setting there is an anaphylaxis kit on every ward, which is usually placed on the crash trolley in a yellow box. You should ensure senior help is available, either by putting out a crash call in a hospital or calling 999 if in the community.

If the patient has signs of respiratory or cardiovascular compromise, immediately give 0.5 mg of adrenaline intramuscularly (0.5 mL 1:1000). Adrenaline will act rapidly (seconds to minutes) with α-adrenergic effects (vasoconstriction) and β-adrenergic effects (bronchial dilation).

Manage the patient using the ABC pathway:

A Airway – Assess that the airway is patent. Call for anaesthetic support if the airway is compromised, and use basic life-support techniques (head tilt, chin lift, jaw thrust).
B Breathing – Auscultate the praecordium and observe the chest wall movement to ensure equal and symmetrical movement. Monitor the respiratory rate and the oxygen saturations. In the acute setting, apply 15 L oxygen via a non-rebreathe mask if the patient is dyspnoeic or desaturating. If you can hear wheeze, administer a bronchodilator, such as a salbutamol nebulizer and a muscarinic agonist, such as an ipratropium bromide nebulizer. Consider doing an arterial blood gas test.
C Circulation – Monitor the heart rate and blood pressure. Tachycardia and hypotension are signs of circulatory compromise. Listen to the patient's heart, check the pulse and the capillary refill time. Ensure the patient has intravenous access with a large-bore cannula. Start intravenous fluids, preferably a colloid if the patient is hypotensive.

Remember that adrenaline acts for a short duration and that its effects may wear off after 15 minutes or so. Consider giving another dose if necessary.

Alongside adrenaline, give 200 mg of hydrocortisone intravenously. This is a corticosteroid that acts to decrease eosinophil action and generally reduce the inflammatory response. Remember that corticosteroids typically take several hours to have a significant effect.

Chlorpheniramine 10 mg intramuscularly should be administered. Chlorpheniramine is a histamine H1 receptor antagonist and can prevent the excess histamine generated in response to an allergen from triggering further immune responses, but also has little effect for over an hour.

The patient will need to be reviewed by a senior doctor and should be monitored closely for a further 24 hours.

Around 1 in 5 patients develop a late-phase anaphylactic reaction 4–8 hours after the initial episode, despite no further exposure to the allergen. This occurs when neutrophils and eosinophils migrate to the site of the initial allergen-recognition and generate a further inflammatory response. Cytokines released from mast cells may remain present for several hours also, provoking ongoing inflammation.

Intravenous fluid rehydration should be continued for 4–6 hours, and the patient will require regular monitoring to review whether she needs further doses of adrenaline and nebulizers.

The patient should be informed that she has had a life-threatening allergic response to a penicillin-based drug and should advise medical staff of this whenever she attends hospital. Her medical records must be updated and her GP informed. An allergy bracelet should be worn during her hospital stay. If there is doubt about the precipitant of the anaphylactic reaction, an allergy clinic referral should be made.

 KEY POINTS

- Always ask a patient about allergies when taking a history. It is vital to know about allergies to medications.
- Anaphylaxis is a medical emergency. Treat the patient immediately with intramuscular adrenaline from the crash trolley and call for help.
- Manage the patient according to the ABC principles. Are your basic life support skills up to date?
- Some combination antibiotics, such as Augmentin (co-amoxiclav) and Tazocin (piperacillin/tazobactam) are penicillin-based, so always check whether the drug contains a penicillin before prescribing it.

CASE 74: CONSTIPATION WITH CONFUSION

History

A 71-year-old man has been brought to hospital by his daughter, in a confused state. He was unable to give any history to the doctors. His daughter has told the staff that he mentioned becoming increasingly constipated over recent weeks but seemed to be well otherwise. He had generalized aches and pains that had been bothering him, but attributed them to arthritis, although his GP had arranged a bone scan (see Fig. 74.1) and protein electrophoresis (see Fig. 74.2) to investigate this further. When she visited him earlier in the day he was lying in bed, distressed and with obvious pain in his left arm. He was orientated to person but not time nor place.

Examination

His blood pressure is 160/94 mmHg and his pulse 102/min, thought to be secondary to pain. An X-ray of his left arm shows a fracture in the mid-shaft of the humerus. The orthopaedics team believe this to be a pathological fracture.

INVESTIGATIONS		
		Normal range
White cells	6.0	$4–11 \times 10^9$/L
Haemoglobin	11.8	13–18 g/dL
Platelets	320	$150–400 \times 10^9$/L
Sodium	138	135–145 mmol/L
Potassium	4.2	3.5–5.0 mmol/L
Urea	14	3.0–7.0 mmol/L
Creatinine	150	60–110 µmol/L
Corrected calcium	3.1	2.2–2.6 mmol/L

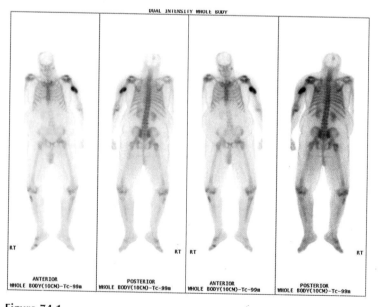

DUAL INTENSITY WHOLE BODY

RT   RT   RT   RT

ANTERIOR
WHOLE BODY(10CM)-Tc-99m

POSTERIOR
WHOLE BODY(10CM)-Tc-99m

ANTERIOR
WHOLE BODY(10CM)-Tc-99m

POSTERIOR
WHOLE BODY(10CM)-Tc-99m

Figure 74.1

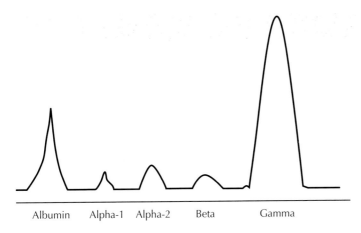

Albumin   Alpha-1   Alpha-2   Beta   Gamma

Figure 74.2

Questions

- What is the most probable underlying diagnosis?
- How could you confirm your suspected diagnosis?
- What treatment should be given to this man in the first 24 hours of his stay?

This man has symptoms of hypercalcaemia ('bones, stones, abdominal groans and psychic moans') and is likely to have multiple myeloma.

Multiple myeloma is a cancer of the plasma cells in the blood, which are responsible for producing antibodies. These abnormal cells form collections in bony spaces (plasmacytomas) which cause lytic lesions and predispose to pathological fractures (i.e. fractures that are unexpected given the history, with no appropriate traumatic cause).

Plasmacytomas can also accumulate in the bone marrow, leading to impaired haematopoesis. Patients present with symptoms related to poor red cell production (pallor, fatigue, shortness of breath, light-headedness), poor white cell production (infections) and poor platelet production (bruising, prolonged bleeding times).

Kidney injury is common in multiple myeloma. This can be secondary to hypercalcaemia but also due to deposition of Bence–Jones proteins that are characteristically produced during myeloma, and damage the renal tubules.

Routine blood tests, checking the full blood count, renal and liver function and a bone profile should be performed. An erythrocyte sedimentation rate (ESR) sample should be taken. A blood film should be sent to look for features of myelodysplasia.

Serum and urine protein electrophoresis will confirm the presence of an abnormal paraprotein band (Fig. 74.2 shows serum electrophoresis with the presence of an abnormally raised gamma band). Urine should be sent to look for Bence–Jones proteins.

The haematology team will usually perform bone marrow aspirate and trephine sampling to confirm the diagnosis.

This patient needs to have his electrolyte imbalances corrected immediately. He will need aggressive fluid rehydration to improve his hypercalcaemia, and intravenous pamidronate, a bisphosphonate, may also be needed to sequester calcium in the bone.

His renal function has acutely deteriorated. This may be due to dehydration and hypercalcaemia, but might be due to renal tubular damage by Bence–Jones protein deposition, as mentioned above. Fluid rehydration may help to improve the renal function. Hyperkalaemia can lead to cardiac arrhythmias; if the potassium level is greater than 6 mmol/L, this should be urgently corrected.

He will need analgesia for his humeral fracture and a referral to the orthopaedics team. Ultimately, a referral to the haematology team will enable complete investigation and long-term management of this man's multiple myeloma.

A bone scan is sometimes carried out to identify areas of bone abnormalities, and in this case there is an abnormal area of myeloma deposition (dark patch) where the humeral fracture was sustained, as well as in the left radius, left and right tibias and occiput. Myelomatous deposits show up better on X-rays and a skeletal survey is usually carried out, where radiographs of the skull, spine, humeri, ribs, pelvis and femurs are performed.

KEY POINTS

- Hypercalcaemia can present with non-specific symptoms such as fatigue, constipation and joint aches.
- Fluid rehydration is the key to improving hypercalcaemia in the presence of malignancy. If fluids are not reducing the calcium levels, bisphosphanates, such as pamidronate, can be used.

CASE 75: CHEST PAIN AFTER EXERTION

History
A 54-year-old man has presented to the emergency department with central, crushing chest pain radiating to his left arm and jaw. The pain came on over 5–10 minutes after he had been running for a bus. He says the pain is 9/10 in severity and is associated with nausea and shortness of breath. His medical history includes hypertension and type 2 diabetes mellitus. He has smoked 20 cigarettes per day for 30 years. His regular medication includes aspirin, ramipril and metformin.

Examination
This man is overweight and visibly uncomfortable. His heart rate is 100/min and blood pressure 140/88 mmHg. He was given 300 mg of aspirin and a glyceryl trinitrate (GTN) spray by the paramedics, which has eased the pain. An ECG was performed, which was normal.

Questions
- What do the symptoms suggest?
- What can be done for this man acutely?

ANSWER 75

The description of the pain is typical for myocardial ischaemia. The pain is central and heavy and radiates to the left arm and jaw. An ECG was performed, which was normal, excluding an ST-elevation myocardial infarction (STEMI). He therefore has acute coronary syndrome (ACS). This could be unstable angina or a non-ST-elevation myocardial infarction (NSTEMI). The definitive test will be a troponin I or T level, which is taken as a blood sample, 12 hours after the onset of chest pain. Troponin is a protein contained in cardiac-muscle thin filaments. Troponin I and troponin T are both sensitive and specific for cardiac damage and can therefore be used as a measure for cardiac infarction. The levels of troponin released into the blood peak after 12 hours, which is when the test is typically carried out.

Begin treatment for ACS immediately, unless there are any contraindications (e.g. if the patient has active bleeding or a history of prolonged bleeding, you may want to consider using standard management). A patient with suspected ACS should be given aspirin, a P2Y12 inhibitor and fundoparinux. Dual antiplatelet therapy is though to reduce further thrombus formation.

GTN will provide nitric oxide that acts on the endothelial smooth muscle to cause vasodilatation. This opens up the coronary blood vessels, allowing more blood and oxygen to reach the cardiac tissue. Oxygen should be given if the patient is short of breath or has low oxygen saturations. In many centres, oxygen is applied routinely in suspected myocardial infarction, although the evidence for this is debatable.

A beta-bocker (e.g. bisoprolol) can be given as this will slow the heart rate and lower the blood pressure, thus reducing the work of the heart.

Adequate analgesia (e.g. morphine) must be given if needed. Relieving his pain should reduce his blood pressure and heart rate and therefore reduce myocardial work.

The patient should be monitored closely and serial ECGs should be taken to look for any ischaemic changes. Twelve hours from when the pain started, a troponin I or T level should be taken. If this is elevated, the patient will need to be managed with reperfusion interventions. If the troponin level is not elevated, he should be investigated by a cardiologist for suspected unstable angina.

 KEY POINTS

- In patients with acute coronary syndrome, there are three possible diagnoses: STEMI, NSTEMI or unstable angina. If the patient does not have ST elevation on the ECG, he/she should be investigated for NSTEMI and unstable angina.
- A troponin T or I level should be taken 12 hours after the pain started, to identify whether myocardial infarction has occurred. Some centres can do rapid cardiac enzyme checks as soon as the patient presents – these are not as specific as troponin levels, but can be useful in initial diagnosis and management.
- ACS treatment should be given to people with suspected myocardial infarction as soon as possible. Think MONA: morphine, oxygen, nitrates and antiplatelet drugs.

History
A 54-year-old woman presented with a two-week history of fevers, weight loss and night sweats. She denied shortness of breath, cough or haemoptysis, but she had been feeling very fatigued and has a poor appetite. She has not travelled abroad in the last five years and has no known tuberculosis contacts. She has never smoked and has only ever worked in an office. There is no significant medical history or family history.

Examination
This woman had cervical, axillary and inguinal lymphadenopathy. The lymph nodes were 2–3 cm in diameter and rubbery in nature. A lymph node biopsy confirmed that the patient had a non-Hodgkin's lymphoma. A chest X-ray is shown in Fig. 76.1.

Initial treatment
She was given a course of chemotherapy and seemed to tolerate it well. Five days later, however, she presents with fevers and a cough productive of yellow sputum. She is found to have a fever of 40.2°C. Her full blood count is checked, as below.

INVESTIGATIONS		
		Normal range
White cells	2.9	4–11 × 10⁹/L
Neutrophils	0.5	2–7 × 10⁹/L
Haemoglobin	11.0	13–18 g/dL
Platelets	154	150–400 × 10⁹/L

Questions
- What does the chest X-ray show, and what is the differential diagnosis for such an appearance?
- What condition has this patient developed as a result of her chemotherapy?

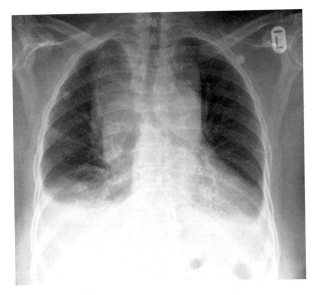

Figure 76.1

ANSWER 76

The chest X-ray shows a widened mediastinum, as well as bilateral pleural effusions and some middle-lobe shadowing. The hila are bulky bilaterally due to lymphadenopathy. There are several disease processes that can cause this appearance:

- primary lung malignancy;
- malignancy with lung metastases;
- lymphoma;
- tuberculosis;
- sarcoidosis.

The patient has presented with a febrile neutropenia (also known as neutropenic sepsis). The chemotherapy has suppressed her bone marrow function and she now has a very low neutrophil count, which puts her at high risk of bacterial infections.

She will need to be started on antibiotics for neutropenic sepsis as per the antibiotic protocol of the individual hospital. She should be started on antibiotics within an hour, as per the Surviving Sepsis guidelines (http://www.survivingsepsis.org). Samples of blood, urine, sputum and stool should be sent for microscopy, culture and sensitivity to attempt to isolate a specific bacterium causing the infection.

Her blood count will need to be monitored at least once a day. Bone marrow suppression can lead to reduced red cell and platelet counts. The haematology team will need to review the patient and may consider giving granulocyte colony-stimulating factor (gCSF) to improve bone marrow function.

She should be nursed in a side room and barrier protection (face masks, gloves and aprons) should be worn when coming into contact with the patient to prevent introducing further sources of infection.

 KEY POINTS

- Chemotherapy can suppress the bone marrow, leading to pancytopenia. A low neutrophil count is strongly associated with increased bacterial infections.
- Neutropenic sepsis is a medical emergency and requires urgent treatment with antibiotics.

CASE 77: RIGHT-SIDED CHEST PAIN

History
A 38-year-old woman has presented to the emergency department with chest pain and shortness of breath. The pain is located around the right side of her chest and is made worse on deep inspiration. The shortness of breath had come on suddenly at rest. She denies any symptoms of cough or fever. Her history is significant for two miscarriages and a deep vein thrombosis (DVT) in her left calf. Apart from the oral contraceptive pill, she does not take any regular medications. Her sister also had a DVT some years ago.

Examination
This woman's chest has good air entry throughout all lung fields with no added sounds. Her calves are soft and non-tender and there is no pitting oedema. Her full blood count and renal function tests are unremarkable. A chest X-ray is normal. Observations: heart rate 94/min, blood pressure 126/82 mmHg, respiratory rate 20/min, SaO_2 94 per cent on room air.

Questions
- What is the differential diagnosis?
- How would you further investigate and manage the patient?

The patient has pleuritic chest pain with shortness of breath. This could be a pneumonia, although you would typically expect symptoms of a cough or fever with a raised white cell count and abnormal findings on examination.

Musculoskeletal injuries can cause pleuritic-type chest pain and, sometimes, shortness of breath, but the patient gives no history of an injury and you would not normally expect low oxygen saturations with such a scenario.

A pulmonary embolus (PE) is the most likely diagnosis. Risk factors for pulmonary embolus include:

- prolonged immobility, such as after surgery or a long-haul flight;
- pregnancy;
- use of oestrogen-containing medications, such as the oral contraceptive pill;
- malignancy;
- thrombophilias, such as factor V Leiden and antiphospholipid syndrome.

Pulmonary emboli are usually preceded by a DVT. This patient has had a DVT, as has her sister, suggesting a genetic cause for her clot. The patient has also had multiple miscarriages. She may have antiphospholipid syndrome, a prothrombotic condition that predisposes patients to arterial and venous blood clots, that classically presents with DVTs, PEs and miscarriages. She also takes the oral contraceptive pill, which further increases her risk of developing clots.

After taking the history and suspecting a PE, you can perform a Wells' score on the patient. A score of 0 equates to a low probability for a PE, while a score of 1–2 equates to a moderate probability for a PE. A score above 3 equates to a high probability for a PE.

A D-dimer blood test can be performed to help guide the diagnosis when there is a low probability for a PE. D-dimer is a fibrin degradation product that can form in the presence of a large blood clot, but can also form with most causes of inflammation, such as an injury, an infection or malignancy. An elevated serum D-dimer level is not of much use diagnostically, but a normal D-dimer level will exclude a PE in the vast majority of cases.

If a patient is suspected to have a PE, an arterial blood gas should be performed to ensure the patient is not hypoxic and oxygen therapy should be given if necessary. Provided that there are no contraindications to anticoagulation, a low-molecular-weight heparin (LMWH), such as enoxaparin, should be given, while you await imaging to confirm the diagnosis.

Imaging tests, such a ventilation–perfusion scan or a CT scan of the pulmonary arteries, can be performed and can confirm whether a patient has a clot present.

If there is a pulmonary embolus, long-term anticoagulation with warfarin or heparin should be given for at least six months to prevent further emboli.

This patient has features of antiphospholipid syndrome and should therefore be investigated further for this condition with blood tests for anticardiolipin IgG and lupus anticoagulant at a later date. Any of the above risk factors for PE should be minimized.

- Consider a pulmonary embolus in a patient with pleuritic chest pain, shortness of breath or haemoptysis, particularly if he/she has any of the risk factors mentioned above.
- A Wells score can help in deciding whether the patient is at low, moderate or high risk for developing a PE.
- A D-dimer test can be performed and is useful in excluding a PE if the levels are normal. A high D-dimer does not mean that the patient has a PE, just that there is some active inflammation.

History

A 30-year-old woman has presented to the emergency department with worsening short-ness of breath, now present on minimal exertion. She is generally fit and well but these symptoms started eight months ago. She is a non-smoker and does not drink alcohol. She takes the combined oral contraceptive pill but no other medications. There are no significant medical problems. There is no history of skin lesions or joint pains. She did complain of fatigue, palpitations and feeling faint. There is no family history of venous thromboembolism or cardiorespiratory problems.

Examination

This woman has no chest pain, cough, swelling of ankles, loss of weight or fever. Cardiovascular examination reveals a left parasternal heave, loud second heart sound with a pansystolic murmur loudest at the left sternal edge. Jugular venous pulse (JVP) shows a prominent V wave. Respiratory and abdominal examinations are unremark-able. There is no clubbing. An ECG is shown in Fig. 78.1. A chest X-ray shows enlarged hilar vessels with an enlarged pulmonary artery shadow. Observations: blood pressure 121/65 mmHg, heart rate 88/min, respiratory rate 25/min, SaO_2 88 per cent on room air.

INVESTIGATIONS		
		Normal range
White cells	8.0	$4–11 \times 10^9$/L
Haemoglobin	15.4	$13–18 \times 10^9$/L
Platelets	198	$150–400 \times 10^9$/L
Sodium	139	135–145 mmol/L
Potassium	3.6	3.5–5.0 mmol/L
Urea	5.8	3.0–7.0 mmol/L
Creatinine	77	60–110 µmol/L

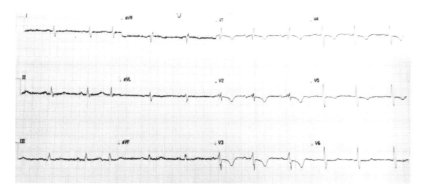

Figure 78.1

Questions

- What is the most likely diagnosis?
- What further investigations would you perform to determine the cause of her symp-toms?
- How would you manage this patient?

The ECG shows right axis deviation, a predominant R wave in lead V1 and inverted T waves in lead V2, which are suggestive of right ventricular hypertrophy. There are also peaked P waves, showing there is a degree of right atrial enlargement. The presence of progressive dyspnoea with these ECG findings, the chest X-ray appearance, and cardiovascular findings indicate that she may have pulmonary hypertension.

Causes of pulmonary hypertension can be classified as:

- idiopathic;
- familial;
- associated with connective tissue disease, congenital systemic to pulmonary shunts, portal hypertension, HIV, drugs and toxins;
- pulmonary veno-occlusive disease;
- pulmonary capillary haemangiomatosis;
- associated with left-sided atrial or ventricular disease or valvular disease;
- associated with respiratory disease (COPD, interstitial lung disease);
- chronic thromboembolic disease;
- other causes: sarcoidosis, lymphangiomatosis, histiocytosis X.

This patient requires further investigations to determine the cause. She is young with no significant past medical history or abnormalities on basic blood tests. She is short of breath and hypoxic, so she needs supplemental oxygen to correct hypoxaemia. The possibility of idiopathic pulmonary hypertension is raised but that is a diagnosis of exclusion. She should undergo an urgent echocardiogram to assess estimated right ventricular systolic pressure as well as right ventricular and atrial size. Assessments of the pulmonary and tricuspid valves can also be performed. She will need to undergo a right heart catheterization to determine the severity of hypertension and rule out other causes. Other tests to be performed include full blood count, liver function, thyroid function, HIV status, ventilation–perfusion scan and antinuclear antibodies (ANA) to help differentiate from the other causes.

Idiopathic pulmonary hypertension (IPH) is defined by a mean pulmonary artery pressure >25 mmHg at rest or >30 mmHg with exercise, without a known cause. It is, however, rare (estimated incidence of 1–2 per million population).

Testing of B-type natriuretic peptide (BNP) gives an indication of right heart strain and correlates with mortality.

Medications that can be used in those with right heart strain include diuretics (if there is fluid retention). Anticoagulation with warfarin is recommended in all patients. Some cases of IPH do respond to vasodilators and do benefit from calcium-channel antagonists such as nifedipine or diltiazem. She should therefore undergo a vasodilator test to see if pulmonary hypertension decreases. She should be managed in a centre that specializes in IPH so that other specific medications can be tried or if necessary she can be considered for lung transplantation.

Medications that have been proven to offer benefit in pulmonary hypertension include vasoactive substances to reduce pulmonary pressures. Infusions of prostacyclin are among the most effective treatments in reducing pulmonary pressures, but are currently not available in oral form. There are several inhaled forms of prostacyclins, the most commonly used being iloprost. Phosphodiesterase 5 inhibitors, such as sildenafil, relax vascular smooth muscle and can also be of benefit in pulmonary hypertension. Bosentan

is an endothelin receptor agonist that blocks endothelin-medilated pulmonary vasoconstriction and is available in a tablet form.

 KEY POINTS

- Prognosis is poor with a five-year survival rate of about 34 per cent.
- Idiopathic pulmonary hypertension is rare and is a diagnosis of exclusion.

History

A 16-year-old girl was found unconscious in her room and has been brought to hospital. She was diagnosed with type 1 diabetes mellitus three years earlier, and currently uses NovoMix 30, 8 units twice daily. Her glycated haemoglobin (HbA1c) was checked last month and was 6.1 per cent (normal range 4–5.9), indicating an average blood glucose level of 7.0 mmol/L over the past three months. She has been suffering from a sore throat and influenza-like symptoms over the preceding days. Her parents say that she has not given herself as much insulin as normal as she had been eating and drinking less.

Examination

Her mucous membranes are dry. Her abdomen is soft but tender throughout. She vomits several times during the examination. She appears short of breath and is gasping. Her blood sugar, checked by the paramedics, is 24 mmol/L. Observations: temperature 36.8°C, heart rate 110/min, blood pressure 90/50 mmHg, respiratory rate 32/min, SaO_2 99 per cent on room air.

INVESTIGATIONS		
		Normal range
Urine dip:		
Glucose	4+	
Ketones	3+	
Arterial blood gas on room air:		
pH	7.12	7.35 –7.45
PO_2	12.8	9.3–13.3 kPa
PCO_2	2.8	4.7–6.0 kPa
Lactate	4.0	<2 mmol/L
HCO_3	18	22–26 mmol/L
Base excess	−6	−3 to +3 mmol/L

Questions
- What is the underlying diagnosis?
- How would you manage this patient acutely?

ANSWER 79

The patient is likely to have diabetic ketoacidosis (DKA). She has not been adhering to her usual insulin regime and is now hyperglycaemic. She has ketones in her urine and the blood gas sample shows a metabolic acidosis (low pH with low HCO_3; the PCO_2 is also low, ruling out any respiratory component to the acidosis).

When people become dehydrated, the body produces stress hormones that increase glucose availability to allow for increased metabolic requirements. When there is a lack of insulin in the body, such as in this case, high levels of glucose are released by the liver from glycogen stores and gluconeogenesis. The kidneys begin to excrete glucose in the urine and via osmosis; this leads to water and electrolytes leaving the body in the urine. The patient experiences polyuria and becomes increasingly dehydrated. Fatty acids are broken down, producing ketones.

The patient is likely to be very dehydrated. The priority should be to correct her fluid status. She should receive a stat 1 L bag of normal saline, which will run in over around 10 minutes. A urinary catheter should be sited to allow proper fluid balance measurements to be recorded. She should be given a further 1–2 L of fluid over the next hour.

An intravenous sliding scale of insulin and fluid should be set up. This means that a short-acting insulin is continuously infused through a pump into the bloodstream. Blood glucose measurements are taken frequently via a finger-prick test and the rate of insulin is adjusted according to the results. Most hospitals have a sliding scale protocol available for this.

Electrolytes, particularly potassium, may need to be corrected, as patients with DKA lose potassium through their urine. Potassium levels will need to be measured hourly at first and can usually be done via a blood gas test.

The acidosis will usually resolve with fluid rehydration and correction of hyperglycaemia. As the insulin levels increase, the fatty acid breakdown will cease and ketones will no longer be produced. If the patient continues to have a low pH, he/she should be taken to a high-dependency setting for closer monitoring and possibly correction of acid–base balance with intravenous sodium bicarbonate solution.

After 24 hours, when the patient is stable and there are no more ketones in the urine, consider stopping the sliding scale and reverting back to the normal insulin regimen. The patient should be educated, ideally by a diabetes nurse specialist, about the importance of maintaining adequate hydration and the importance of regular blood glucose monitoring at home to allow insulin to be titrated accordingly.

 KEY POINTS

- Diabetic ketoacidosis is a life-threatening condition and should be treated urgently.
- The priority is to rehydrate the patient, then correct the high glucose level. You may also need to replace potassium. Monitor the patient's pH, blood glucose and potassium level frequently. If the pH is very low, the patient may need acid–base correction and will require close monitoring.
- If the patient does not respond to treatment within the first 2 hours, he/she should be moved to a high-dependency setting.

History

A 52-year-old man complained of a dull ache in his chest, while sitting down after a meal. He described the pain as being like indigestion but it worsened over the next 30 minutes. His wife noticed that he was looking pale and clammy. He felt the pain radiate to his jaw and left arm. His wife called an ambulance and he arrived in the emergency department about 50 minutes after the pain started. An ECG was performed in the ambulance (see Fig. 80.1) and he was given morphine, glycerine trinitrate spray, aspirin and clopidogrel. He is a smoker of 20 cigarettes daily for 27 years. He is on treatment for hypertension and hypercholesterolaemia. He is not diabetic. His brother had a heart attack at the age of 60 years.

Examination

On arrival at the emergency department he was clammy and in pain. His cardiovascular, respiratory and abdominal examinations were unremarkable. His blood pressure was 159/85 mmHg and heart rate regular at 92/min. An ECG still showed the previous findings. He was taken to the cardiac angiography suite for a coronary angiogram (see Fig. 80.2), when he was also given intravenous heparin.

Treatment

He was treated with a coronary stent and admitted to the coronary care unit. He remained stable with no further chest pain and with resolution of his ECG changes. An echocardiogram performed a few days later showed a good-sized left ventricle with overall preserved systolic function. No regional wall motion abnormalities or valvular dysfunction were reported. He was able to mobilize without further pain and was discharged home after five days.

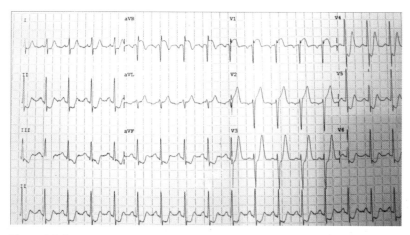

Figure 80.1

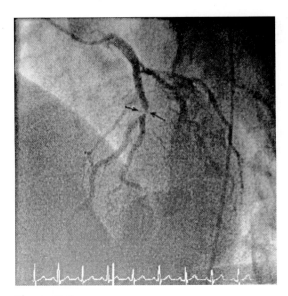

Figure 80.2

Questions
- What is the diagnosis?
- What should be the initial management of this presentation?
- What complications can arise during the next few days?
- Are there any issues for this man's cardiac rehabilitation?

ANSWER 80

This man has had an anterior ST-elevation myocardial infarction (STEMI). The working diagnosis is based on his symptoms of chest pain that is characteristic of 'cardiac' pain and ECG findings. At this stage there will be no markers of myocardial necrosis (troponins) available. In his past medical history he does describe worsening exertional angina of recent onset with risk factors that indicate he is at high risk of cardiovascular events. His angiogram in Fig. 80.2 demonstrates a short stenosis in the mid left anterior descending coronary artery prior to the diagonal branch (arrows).

The diagnosis must be made as quickly as possible. An initial assessment is made in the ambulance ensuring haemodynamic stability. Early reperfusion of the occluded coronary artery is the mainstay of treatment. In this case an ECG performed in the ambulance can result in early diagnosis and transfer to a hospital capable of percutaneous coronary intervention (PCI). Primary PCI should be performed within 2 hours of the first ECG diagnosis. If there is going to be a delay to this then fibrinolytic therapy should be administered.

This man was transferred to a hospital that was able to perform PCI within the recommended time period. He also received antiplatelet agents – aspirin and clopidogrel including heparin in the catheter suite. The blocked artery was identified and re-opened with a coronary stent.

Other treatments that should be started as soon as the patient is stable include a beta-blocker. An oral angiotensin-converting enzyme (ACE) inhibitor should also be given on the first day in patients with significant LV dysfunction. Statins also should be initiated to achieve a low-density lipoprotein (LDL) cholesterol <2 mmol/L.

Complications include pump failure causing cardiogenic shock, rupture of the mitral valve chordae tendinae and perforation of the myocardial wall (septal or free wall) and arrhythmias. Echocardiography can help to distinguish these complications. This man had an uneventful recovery and his echocardiogram demonstrated that he has not had any significant myocardial damage.

Cardiac rehabilitation should focus on medications and lifestyle changes (smoking cessation, diet and exercise). An important area to discuss is the patient's occupation. The Driver and Vehicle Licensing Agency (DVLA) has strict criteria for drivers. Current rules are that STEMI sufferers cannot drive for at least six weeks and must undergo an exercise test or other functional testing to demonstrate there is no further ischaemia.

 KEY POINTS

- Making a swift diagnosis of an ST-elevation myocardial infarction is essential.
- Early reperfusion of the coronary arteries will save cardiac muscle and preserve heart function.

History

A 22-year-old man has been brought by ambulance to the emergency department after his girlfriend found him unconscious at home. She says that he is a regular heroin user. She found him with a needle and syringe in his hand but is unsure what he had injected himself with. He has no medical or surgical history.

Examination

This young man is drowsy but rousable. His pupils are very small. His respiratory rate is 6/min but his lungs sound clear. He has needle track marks up his arm, as well as a fresh puncture mark in the left antecubital fossa.

Questions

- How can this patient's consciousness level be assessed?
- What is the likely cause of the reduced consciousness?
- How would you manage this patient?

ANSWER 81

There are two main scoring systems used for assessing a patient's consciousness level: the AVPU and the GCS.

The AVPU score is based on noting whether the patient is:

A Alert spontaneously;
V alert to Voice;
P alert to Pain;
U Unresponsive.

Although the system is not very detailed, it does allow you to very rapidly note how responsive a patient is and often prompts you to take action and call for help if the patient is scoring a V or less.

The second commonly used scoring system is the Glasgow Coma Scale (see Table 81.1). Patients score points for their verbal response, whether their eyes are open, and the movements that they make. The GCS is an objective score that allows a patient's neurological function to be accurately assessed and monitored.

Table 81.1 Scoring on the Glasgow Coma Scale

GCS score	Best eye response (E)	Best verbal response (V)	Best motor response (M)
1	Does not open eyes	Makes no sounds	Makes no movements
2	Eyes open to pain	Incomprehensible sounds	Extension to painful stimuli (decerebrate response)
3	Eyes open to voice	Inappropriate words	Abnormal flexion to painful stimuli (decorticate response)
4	Eyes open spontaneously	Confused	Flexes/withdraws from painful stimuli
5	–	Orientated, normal conversation	Localizes painful stimuli
6	–	–	Moves obeying commands

The patient has a history of substance misuse, and from the examination it can be concluded that he has injected himself with something, probably heroin. Like morphine, heroin is an opiate drug and features of opiate toxicity are manifold.

- *Respiratory system.* There is a slow respiratory rate with shallow breathing. This can progress to respiratory arrest.
- *Abdominal system.* Vomiting is common and, if the patient has a reduced consciousness level, there is a risk of aspirating (inhaling) the vomit. Later, once the patient has recovered, he/she is likely to be constipated, as the opiate drug will slow intestinal motility.
- *Neurological system.* Patients show a reduced consciousness level and may be unable to protect the airway. They may present anywhere on a spectrum from alert and orientated, to confused and drowsy, to comatose. A classic sign of opiate toxicity is small pupils, which are often described as 'pin-point'.

The first thing to do is assess the patient according to the ABCD protocol. Then a scoring system should be applied. For example, a GCS score of 8 or less means that the patient is probably not able to safely protect his/her own airway, so simple airway management techniques should be carried out until a senior doctor or member of the anaesthetics team can assess for more definitive airway management.

Naloxone is an opiate antagonist and can be used to reverse the effects of morphine and heroin. Naloxone acts within seconds and patients will often dramatically regain consciousness, but the drug effect lasts only for a few minutes. An infusion of naloxone may need to be given; ideally this would be done in a high-dependency setting.

KEY POINTS

- In any patient with a reduced consciousness level, a neurological scoring system should be applied. This allows monitoring of improvement or deterioration in consciousness.
- Signs of opiate overdose include reduced consciousness level, pin-point pupils, reduced respiratory rate and vomiting.
- With a suspected opiate overdose, help from senior doctors should be sought as the patient may need to be managed in a high-dependency setting.

CASE 82: STEADY DETERIORATION IN FUNCTION

History

A 55-year-old man has been brought into the emergency department by his wife because he has been deteriorating over the last three months. Initially she noticed him becoming confused and forgetful. Then he started to become unsteady and uncoordinated. He developed problems with walking and now has trouble swallowing, has slurred speech, very slow movements and occasional jerks. He smokes about 15 cigarettes per day and drinks a glass of wine most days with his meal. He is not on regular medications. There is no family history of similar problems.

Examination

Cardiovascular, respiratory and gastrointestinal examinations are unremarkable. A neurological examination shows no limb weakness but there is increased upper-limb tone, and a coarse, pill-rolling tremor. He is unable to complete an abbreviated mental test. He is noted to have myoclonus and a rigid posture. A CT head scan is described as normal. An MRI was performed which shows hyperintensity in the cerebral cortex and thalamus on diffusion-weighted imaging and fluid-attenuated inversion recovery. An EEG shows periodic spike-wave complexes. Observations: temperature 36°C, blood pressure 142/85 mmHg, heart rate 78/min, respiratory rate 20/min.

INVESTIGATIONS		
		Normal range
White cells	5.1	4–11 × 10⁹/L
Haemoglobin	14.0	13–18 g/dL
Platelets	250	150–400 × 10⁹/L
Sodium	135	135–145 mmol/L
Potassium	4.2	3.5–5.0 mmol/L
Urea	7.0	3.0–7.0 mmol/L
Creatinine	110	60–110 µmol/L
C-reactive protein	<5	<5 mg/L
Bilirubin	12	5–25 µmol/L
Alanine aminotransferase	21	8–55 IU/L
Alkaline phosphatase	85	42–98 IU/L
Albumin	39	35–50 g/L
Thyroid-stimulating hormone	3.2	0.4–3.5 mIU/L
Venereal Disease Research Laboratory (VDRL) test	Negative	
Lyme disease	Negative	
HIV	Negative	
Antinuclear antibodies	Negative	
Antinuclear cytoplasmic antibodies	Negative	

Questions

- What is the most likely diagnosis?
- What additional investigations would be helpful?

This man has a rapidly progressive dementia with primarily parkinsonian abnormalities. The differential diagnoses include Alzheimer's disease (tends to be more chronic in onset), Lewy body dementia (similar presentation with parkinsonian features), frontotemporal dementia, cerebral vasculitis, paraneoplastic and non-paraneoplastic limbic encephalitis, and other infections (HIV, syphilis). However, with the MRI and EEG findings, history and initial blood tests, sporadic Creutzfeldt–Jakob disease (sCJD) is likely.

The most helpful investigation is MRI, as specific changes in the thalamus on DWI and FLAIR sequences are strongly suggestive of sCJD. Other tests to rule out infectious, toxic, malignant or vasculitic processes should be guided by the history and examination. Ultimately a brain biopsy is the only definitive way to diagnose CJD. However, this is rarely performed. There can be a false-negative result as prion accumulation occurs at variable places.

Sporadic CJD has no cure. Treatment is supportive with the aim to control myoclonus, agitation and mood disturbances.

CJD is classified as sporadic, familial or acquired (variant CJD from consumption of beef contaminated with bovine spongiform encephalopathy). The sporadic form is the most common and is idiopathic. It is characterized by a progressive dementia with either pyramidal or extrapyramidal weakness, myoclonus, visual or cerebellar disturbance or akinetic mutism with characteristic EEG findings.

The causative agent of CJD is prion protein. Misfolded prions act as templates to cause other prions nearby to misfold. They rapidly accumulate in nerve cells, causing cellular death and spongiform appearance of brain tissue.

 KEY POINTS

- Creutzfeldt–Jakob disease is a prion disease that is very rare but always fatal.
- CJD often presents similarly to other disease processes, but MRI and EEG are helpful in supporting the diagnosis. Ultimately, if required, a brain biopsy will provide a definitive diagnosis.

CASE 83: EXACERBATION OF COPD

History
A 66-year-old woman has presented with shortness of breath and a cough. She has been feeling unwell for a week, with a cough productive of green sputum. She is known to have chronic obstructive pulmonary disease (COPD) and has had multiple previous hospital admissions with infective exacerbations. She is on treatment with inhaled bronchodilators and inhaled corticosteroids. She gave up smoking two years ago.

Examination
This woman is visibly dyspnoeic with a respiratory rate of 40/min. She has an end-expiratory wheeze throughout all lung fields and coarse crackles at the right lung base. On presentation her oxygen saturations were 84 per cent on room air, but after being given 2 L/min oxygen via a Hudson mask the saturations increased to 96 per cent. Arterial blood gas results are shown below.

INVESTIGATIONS			
	Room air	2 L/min O_2	Normal range
pH	7.42	7.31	7.35–7.45
PO_2	7.0	9.0	9.3–13.3 kPa
PCO_2	6.6	8.0	4.7–6.0 kPa
Lactate	1.0	2.1	<2 mmol/L
HCO_3	24	26	22–26 mmol/L
Base excess	+1	+3	−3 to +3 mmol/L
Saturation	84%	96%	>94%

Questions
- This patient is having an infective exacerbation of COPD. How will you treat her initially?
- Interpret the blood gas results and suggest treatment options.

The patient will need broad-spectrum antibiotics; whether they are given orally or intravenously will depend on the patient's clinical status and her blood results. In this case, the patient is unwell and will probably need intravenous antibiotics for at least 24 hours. A sputum sample should be taken and sent for microscopy, culture and sensitivity so that targeted antibiotic therapy can later be given. If possible, try to find out whether the patient has previously grown any specific bacteria in her sputum as this may guide antibiotic choice.

Prescribe bronchodilating nebulizers, starting with salbutamol, a B_2 agonist, which will help to open up the airways. Nebulized ipratropium bromide, an anticholinergic, should also be given to block the smooth muscle acetylcholine receptors in the bronchi.

A course of steroids should be commenced, usually oral prednisolone for 7–10 days. This will dampen down the inflammatory response in the airways.

She will need an oxygen prescription chart, stating her target saturations, to inform the ward staff of how much oxygen to give her at any point in time and when to call for a doctor to review her oxygen requirements.

An arterial blood gas sample should always be performed on room air, to assess for hypoxia and hypercapnia. In this case, the patient had a blood gas on admission and a repeat test after oxygen was administered. The arterial blood gas may need to be repeated if a different concentration of oxygen is given or if her clinical condition changes.

If the patient's condition fails to improve, other drugs (e.g. the bronchodilator aminophylline) may be needed. If this is the case, the high-dependency unit should be notified, as she may need to be transferred to a ward with a higher level of care.

The first blood gas shows that the patient is hypoxic with a low PO_2. The second blood gas shows that, although her oxygen saturations and PO_2 have picked up with 2 L/min oxygen, her PCO_2 has increased and she now has a metabolic acidosis. She has a low PO_2 and a high PCO_2 – this is type 2 respiratory failure.

Due to chronic impaired gas exchange, this woman probably always has a high baseline PCO_2, which means that her hypercapnic drive has been blunted over time. In this situation, by improving her PO_2 levels, you will reverse her hypoxic pulmonary vasoconstriction that leads to ineffective CO_2 excretion. Coupled with the Haldane effect, this would result in the further elevation of pCO_2 and thence CO_2 narcosis.

The patient will probably need non-invasive ventilation (NIV) to provide oxygen and help reduce her hypercapnia. She should be transferred to a high-dependency unit or a ward that manages NIV. She will need frequent arterial blood gas measurements to titrate the settings of the NIV.

The patient should have a 'respiratory passport' produced when she has improved, documenting her baseline arterial blood gas results and stating that she is prone to type 2 respiratory failure when given oxygen. Aim for the patient to have oxygen saturations of 88–92 per cent rather than >94 per cent as she can probably tolerate lower oxygen saturations. She should be reviewed by a COPD nurse for future management.

History

A 69-year-old woman has presented to the emergency department with a three-month history of general malaise, loss of appetite and 4 kg loss of weight. She also has sinusitis and a purulent nasal discharge and nose bleeds. She has presented now because of new symptoms of feeling short of breath on exertion and coughing up blood. She has developed painful joints, starting in the wrists but now affecting her ankles and knees.

Examination

This woman looks fatigued and unwell. She has joint swelling on her wrists and ankles with some warmth and tenderness and restricted movement. There is a palpable purpuric rash over her shins. The cardiovascular, respiratory, abdominal and neurological examinations are unremarkable. A chest X-ray shows bilateral pulmonary infiltrates (see Fig. 84.1). Observations: temperature 37.9°C, heart rate 101/min, respiratory rate 28/min, SaO_2 90 per cent on room air.

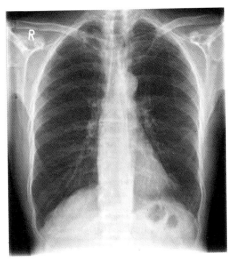

Figure 84.1

INVESTIGATIONS		
		Normal range
White cells	16.0	$4-11 \times 10^9$/L
Neutrophils	14.5	$2-7 \times 10^9$/L
Haemoglobin	9.8	13–18 g/dL
Platelets	580	$150-400 \times 10^9$/L
Sodium	135	135–145 mmol/L
Potassium	6.8	3.5–5.0 mmol/L
Urea	39.2	3.0–7.0 mmol/L
Creatinine	745	60–110 µmol/L
Arterial gas sample on room air:		
pH	7.21	7.35–7.45
PO_2	7.4	9.3–13.3 kPa
PCO_2	4.8	4.7–6.0 kPa
Lactate	3.6	<2 mmol/L
HCO_3	14	22–26 mmol/L
Base excess	−6	−3 to +3 mmol/L
Urine dipstick:		
Protein	2+	
Blood	3+	
Urine microscopy	>100 red blood cells, red cell casts	

Questions

- What is the likely diagnosis and how would you confirm this
- How would you manage this patient?

ANSWER 84

This woman presents with features suggesting a pulmonary–renal syndrome. The systemic signs and a purpuric rash are suggestive of an active vasculitis. In this case the nasal symptoms indicate involvement of the upper respiratory tract, a useful clue to suggest that Wegener's granulomatosis rather than the other vasculitides associated with pulmonary–renal syndromes is the most likely cause.

The diagnosis is based on detecting antineutrophil cytoplasmic antibodies (ANCA) and a biopsy, usually renal, showing active vasculitis. A negative ANCA test can occur in up to 50 per cent of patients with renal involvement. Wegener's granulomatosis is a systemic vasculitis affecting small and medium-sized vessels. Granulomatous inflammation can be observed on biopsy specimens. Renal biopsy shows a pauci-immune glomerulonephritis (few or no immune deposits). It can affect any organ but is most often associated with the respiratory tract and kidneys. The average age of onset is between 40 and 60 years. It affects men and women equally and is predominantly seen in Caucasian people.

Other tests to help confirm the diagnosis can involve a CT of the chest to identify pulmonary infiltrates or cavitating lesions. A raised transfer factor K_{CO} on lung function testing indicates recent pulmonary haemorrhage. Biopsies from affected areas such as upper respiratory tract (granulomatous inflammation, necrosis and vasculitis) and skin (leukocytoclastic vasculitis) may also be helpful.

Acute management includes treating her hypoxia with oxygen. If hypoxia does not improve, intubation may be necessary. She also has acute renal failure with hyperkalaemia and acidosis. Both are life-threatening complications and she should be managed in a high-dependency or intensive-care setting. Untreated Wegener's granulomatosis has a poor prognosis with median survival of only five months. Early involvement of a renal specialist is important to diagnose and treat the underlying condition. First-line therapy is similar to treating Goodpasture's syndrome with pulmonary involvement and includes pulsed methylprednisolone (followed by oral prednisolone) and cyclophosphamide. Plasmapheresis is also required if there is severe organ involvement (respiratory failure requiring ventilatory support, creatinine >354 µmol/L or not responding to first-line therapy). Second-line agents include mycophenolate mofetil, rituximab or leflunamide.

Corticosteroids are continued for one month before weaning. Long-term use of corticosteroids can cause osteoporosis, so supplementation with calcium and vitamin D and addition of a bisphosphonate is required. It is important to provide prophylaxis against *Pneumocystis jiroveci* with strong immunosuppressants. Most patients are given trimethoprim/sulfamethoxazole (160 mg/800 mg orally once daily on alternate days).

Once remission is induced, cyclophosphamide can be switched to azathioprine or methotrexate with further weaning of steroid dose if possible.

Cyclophosphamide can cause infertility in men and women. Long-term follow-up is required with a renal specialist to monitor disease activity and drug side-effects.

 KEY POINTS

- Wegener's granulomatosis has a poor prognosis and must be treated early and aggressively.
- A renal biopsy is required for diagnosis as ANCA may not be positive in up to 50 per cent of cases involving the kidneys.

History

A 56-year-old woman has presented to the emergency department after collapsing at work. She was sitting at her desk when she developed a severe ache at the back of her head. This was so excruciating that she passed out. Witnesses did not note any shaking of limbs, and she came around within a minute. She vomited twice en route to the hospital and complained of double vision. Her medical history includes polycystic kidney disease and hypertension. She is taking ramipril and bendroflumethiazide for hypertension. She does not smoke or drink alcohol. Her sister also has polycystic kidney disease. She did experience a similar but much less severe headache two weeks ago but put it down to strain from using a new work computer.

Examination

This woman is oriented, moving her limbs and speaking appropriately. On neurological examination there is no limb weakness, and reflexes are present and symmetrical. Plantar responses are flexor. She has a ptosis on the left with the eye depressed and abducted. The pupil is dilated and unreactive to light. There is some mild neck stiffness and photophobia. Her cardiorespiratory and abdominal examinations are unremarkable. Observations: temperature 36.4°C, blood pressure 162/85 mmHg, heart rate 78/min, respiratory rate 18/min, SaO_2 98 per cent on room air.

INVESTIGATIONS

		Normal range
White cells	4.0	$4–11 \times 10^9$/L
Haemoglobin	12.1	13–18 g/dL
Platelets	220	$150–400 \times 10^9$/L
Sodium	141	135–145 mmol/L
Potassium	5.0	3.5–5.0 mmol/L
Urea	6	3.0–7.0 mmol/L
Creatinine	98	60–110 µmol/L

Questions

- What is the diagnosis and how might you confirm this?
- What would be the appropriate management?

This woman presents with a sudden onset of a severe occipital headache with evidence of a third nerve palsy, as shown by the ptosis and eye position. Sudden severe headache is characteristic of subarachnoid haemorrhage (SAH). and the third nerve palsy suggests damage to the nerve secondary to rupture of a posterior communicating artery berry aneurysm on the left side. She also has features of mild meningeal irritation and vomiting which can occur in significant bleeds. There is no suggestion of an infective or vasculitic process as her history is acute, she is afebrile and has normal inflammatory markers.

An urgent CT head scan is required to determine the presence of subarachnoid blood, which will show up as hyperdense areas in the basal cisterns possibly extending to the fissures and sulci. Oedema and mass effects may also be detected. With small bleeds, a CT scan can fail to show up blood in the basal cisterns. In this case a lumbar puncture for cerebrospinal fluid (CSF) sampling must be performed. It is recommended that a lumbar puncture be performed after 12 hours from the onset of headache since, if red blood cells are present in the CSF, they will start to break down releasing enough bilirubin and oxy-haemoglobin into the CSF to be detected. It is important to take four samples and to send them to the laboratory immediately, protected from light (which causes oxyhaemoglobin to form more quickly). The laboratory will spin the samples down to ensure no blood cells contaminate the analysis, which might have come from a 'traumatic' tap. Once spun down the CSF can be visually inspected. In significant bleeds the CSF can appear yellow which is the xanthochromia from the bilirubin and oxyhaemoglobin; however, this is not a reliable confirmation and spectrophotometry should be performed which reliably detects the presence of these pigments. It is no longer appropriate to send three consecutive samples to detect a decrease in the number of red cells.

Further assessment involves identifying the cause of the bleed. In this woman a berry aneurysm is suspected. The most common next investigation would be either a CT angiography or MR angiography. They are non-invasive methods, but the gold standard method is catheter angiography.

Most subarachnoid haemorrhages (80 per cent) are caused by the rupture of a saccular aneurysm. They occur at the bifurcations of arteries. Their formation is associated with adult polycystic kidney disease, Marfan syndrome, neurofibromatosis type 1, Ehlers–Danlos syndrome and pseudoxanthomata elasticum.

In this case the patient has a history of polycystic kidney disease (PKD). The most common type is autosomal dominant PKD of which there are two defective genes (PKD1, 80 per cent of cases, and PKD2, 20 per cent). Hypertension is common and chronic renal failure develops by the age of 70 years in those with PKD1. If there is a family history of SAH, the likelihood of SAH in autosomal dominant PKD is much higher than if there is no history of SAH.

If a CT head scan confirms a bleed, the main priorities in acute care are to ensure the patient is stable and to arrange urgent referral to a neurosurgical unit. In this case the patient's Glasgow Coma Scale score is 15/15, but she has neurological signs and her GCS must be monitored frequently to detect any deterioration in consciousness level that might necessitate airway protection. A frequent full neurological examination should also be part of management to detect progression of symptoms, which might indicate further bleeding, oedema or hydrocephalus. She should therefore be managed in an intensive-care unit. She should be started on nimodipine, which prevents vasospasm and has been shown to improve outcomes after aneurysmal bleeds. Strong analgesia should be given for the headache. Hyponatraemia can develop with SAH and abnormal clotting can exacerbate the bleed; hence both must be monitored and corrected.

Urgent referral for surgical intervention to treat a suspected aneurysm is required. The two main methods are either surgical clipping or endovascular coil embolization.

 KEY POINTS

- In suspected subarachnoid haemorrhage, a CT head scan can be normal.
- A lumbar puncture should be performed at least 12 hours after the onset of headache.
- Those with SAH and polycystic kidney disease should warrant screening for cerebral aneurysms in other family members with PKD.

History

A 62-year-old woman presented to her GP worried that she has become increasingly fatigued over the last 18 months and recently her appetite has been poor. She put this down to stress and difficulty coping at home since her retirement. However, her daughter is anxious that she seems to be looking more yellow over the past few weeks. The woman also complains of an itchy sensation making her scratch all the time. She finds she has to drink more water because of a dry mouth. She has not had any abdominal pains, malaena, change in bowel habit or loss of weight. She has hypothyroidism and takes thyroxine replacement, and her sister also has thyroid disease. She does not smoke or drink alcohol. She takes no treatment other than thyroxine.

Examination

This woman looks jaundiced. Xanthelasmas are noted around the eyes. There are spider naevi around her upper torso and arms, and palmar erythema on her hands. Her cardiovascular and respiratory examinations are normal, but in the abdomen she has a mass in the right upper quadrant. No other masses or abnormalities are noted. She is fully orientated and responds appropriately. There is no tremor. Observations: temperature 36.2°C, heart rate 68/min, blood pressure 134/72 mmHg.

INVESTIGATIONS		
		Normal range
White cells	9.1	$4-11 \times 10^9$/L
Haemoglobin	13.0	13–18 g/dL
Platelets	320	$150-400 \times 10^9$/L
Sodium	139	135–145 mmol/L
Potassium	4.0	3.5–5.0 mmol/L
Urea	5.1	3.0–7.0 mmol/L
Creatinine	84	60–110 µmol/L
Bilirubin	154	5–25 µmol/L
Alanine aminotransferase	75	8–55 IU/L
Alkaline phosphatase	834	42–98 IU/L
Gamma-glytamyl transpeptidase	876	8–78 IU/L
Albumin	30	35–50 g/L
INR	1.5	0.9–1.1
Total cholesterol	8.2	3–5 mmol/L

Questions

- What is the likely diagnosis?
- What additional tests would you require to confirm this?
- How would you manage this woman?

ANSWER 86

This woman presents with a chronic pattern of non-specific ill-health with deterioration over the last few weeks, showing jaundice and abnormal liver function tests. The pattern of abnormality suggests an obstructive picture, and the findings suggest primary biliary cirrhosis (PBC). However, other causes of cholestasis should be considered. Antimitochondrial antibody and antinuclear antibody (ANA nuclear ring staining) are present in PBC. The diagnosis is confirmed by a liver biopsy. This shows bile duct cell disruption within inflamed portal tracts and granuloma formation. In more advanced cases there will be loss of bile ducts and biliary fibrosis. In 10 per cent of cases there is a predominantly inflammatory hepatitis pattern. These cases also tend to have elevated IgG levels.

PBC affects predominantly women (10:1) in their late 40s to 60s. It is an autoimmune condition and is associated with other autoimmune syndromes such as Sjögren's syndrome, autoimmune thyroid disease and coeliac disease.

PBC can present asymptomatically and be found only by an abnormal liver biochemistry. Characteristic findings include a raised alkaline phosphatase (ALP) and gamma-GT but only mildy raised or normal transaminases. Another presentation is with non-specific symptoms over several months to years, as in this case. Sometimes patients present with advanced liver disease with evidence of cirrhosis, portal hypertension and jaundice.

This woman has presented to her GP with signs and symptoms of advanced liver disease. She requires urgent admission to hospital for further investigations and management. An initial assessment shows she is not systemically unwell and is haemodynamically stable. There are no significant derangements of electrolytes. Her main liver biochemistry shows a cholestatic picture, so another cause for obstruction to biliary flow must be excluded. In most cases this will involve an ultrasound of the liver, pancreas and biliary/hepatic ducts. The differentials for this woman's presentation would be malignancy involving the bile ducts, head of pancreas or liver, drug-induced cholestasis, primary sclerosing cholangitis (associated with inflammatory bowel disease), and cholangitis (likely to present with systemic signs of sepsis and abdominal pain).

PBC has been shown to respond to ursodeoxycholic acid therapy. If the disease process is diagnosed early, regular treatment can slow further deterioration. If the histology shows an inflammatory component, prednisolone can be used. The level of IgG can gauge the effect of prednisolone. In this case biopsy is likely to show end-stage liver disease. She should be screened with oesophagogastroduodenoscopy (OGD) for varices, which have the potential to bleed. Liver transplantation is an option for those with end-stage liver disease, so in this case discussion with a transplant centre would be the next step.

 KEY POINTS

- Cholesterol is often raised in primary biliary cirrhosis. Statin therapy is not contraindicated.
- Primary biliary cirrhosis presents with a cholestatic picture whereas autoimmune hepatitis mainly affects transaminases – athough there can be a degree of crossover between the two conditions. A liver biopsy can be helpful in distinguishing them.

CASE 87: ABDOMINAL PAIN, BRUISING AND CONFUSION

History

A 48-year-old woman has presented to the emergency department feeling generally unwell with abdominal pain, bruising and confusion. Her husband states that she has been complaining of general tiredness, nausea and joint pains for several months. She has a history of type 1 diabetes and hypothyroidism. She does not smoke or drink alcohol. There has been no exposure to hepatitis or recent travel abroad. Her only prescribed drugs are levothyroxine and insulin and she has not taken any over-the-counter medications.

Examination

This woman appears unwell with deep yellow sclerae, scratch marks, bruising over her arms and legs and spider naevi over her chest and back. There is a coarse tremor of her outstretched hands. In her abdomen there is hepatomegaly and evidence of ascites.

INVESTIGATIONS		
		Normal range
White cells	10.0	4–11 × 10⁹/L
Haemoglobin	10.1	13–18 g/dL
Platelets	208	150–400 × 10⁹/L
Sodium	130	135–145 mmol/L
Potassium	4.5	3.5–5.0 mmol/L
Urea	12	3.0–7.0 mmol/L
Creatinine	140	60–110 µmol/L
Bilirubin	110	5–25 µmol/L
Alanine aminotransferase	4454	8–55 IU/L
Alkaline phosphatase	378	42–98 IU/L
Albumin	28	35–50 g/L
INR	2.8	0.9–1.1

Questions

- What is the diagnosis, and how would you manage this patient?
- What tests would you do to identify the underlying cause?

This woman presents with evidence of hepatic encephalopathy, jaundice and coagulopathy. She is in fulminant hepatic failure. She requires immediate transfer to the intensive-care unit for optimal management and prevention of further complications such as renal failure, cerebral oedema, sepsis and gastrointestinal bleeding. She is at risk of a rapid decline in consciousness if encephalopathy worsens and may need intubation to protect her airway if this occurs. She requires invasive monitoring in the form of central venous and arterial lines to help provide optimal intravascular filling and electrolyte replacements. Blood glucose should be monitored regularly as hypoglycaemia can occur.

Discussion with a tertiary referral centre for liver transplantation should be made. The decision for liver transplantation can be very difficult and is based on the probability of spontaneous hepatic recovery. Various criteria exist to guide decisions on transplantation. For instance, the King's College Hospital criteria include a prothrombin time of >100 seconds (independent of grade of encephalopathy) or any three of the following: age <10 or >40; aetiology (non-A, non-B hepatitis, halothane hepatitis, idiosyncratic drug reactions); duration of jaundice before onset of encephalopathy >7 days; prothrombin time >50 seconds; bilirubin >308 µmol/L.

Identifying the cause of hepatic failure is important as it can determine further therapy and also the likelihood of suitability for liver transplantation. There are several causes of fulminant liver failure, which include viral (hepatitis A, B and D), idiosyncratic (coumarins, carbamezepin, valproic acid, halogenated hydrocarbons), toxins (paracetamol, isoniazid, methotrexate, *Amanita phalloides* toxin), metabolic (Wilson's disease), and vascular (Budd–Chiari syndrome).

In this case she has features suggesting that autoimmune hepatitis (AIH) could be the underlying cause. Blood tests that can help diagnose AIH include anti-SLA/LP (anti-soluble liver antigens or liver/pancreas). These are highly specific for type 1 AIH. Other tests include anti-SMA, and anti-LKM-1 (positive in type 2 AIH). Liver biopsy is essential to establish the diagnosis and determine severity but can be problematic if there is impaired clotting function. The liver is involved with the modification and production of clotting factors, such as vitamin K. Hepatic failure can lead to impaired clotting (as seen in this case, where the patient has an elevated INR and signs of bruising). The characteristic finding is periportal lesions or interface hepatitis (portal mononuclear and plasma cell infiltrate). Panacinar hepatitis and centrilobular necrosis can also be features in AIH.

Treatment for autoimmune hepatitis involves corticosteroids and immunosuppressants. Treatment is recommended for those with serum aminotransferase levels greater than 10-fold the upper limit of normal, or greater than 5-fold upper limit of normal if gamma-globulin is at least twice the upper limit of normal. If histology shows bridging necrosis or multi-acinar necrosis, treatment is recommended also; combination therapy with prednisolone and azathioprine is given. In fulminant hepatic failure, monotherapy with prednisolone (60 mg once daily) can be given with or without consideration for transplant.

AIH can present insidiously with months of mild abdominal discomfort, pruritus, arthralgia and general malaise. It has a poor prognosis with a five-year survival rate of 50 per cent following diagnosis and 10 per cent at 10 years. Liver transplantation in AIH is associated with a five-year patient survival of between 80 and 90 per cent. In some cases AIH can recur in transplanted livers.

KEY POINTS

- Fulminant hepatic failure requires intensive care and discussion with a liver transplant centre.
- AIH can present in a variety of ways: asymptomatic with raised aminotransferases but no fibrosis, or inflammation found on biopsy, to the rare presentation of acute hepatic failure.

History

A 45-year-old man has been referred to the medical admissions unit with a two-week history of fever, malaise and myalgia, having developed central chest discomfort four days ago. He describes the pain as tight, and he was becoming more short of breath on exertion. He has a history of hypertension. He is not on any medications and has no significant family history. He smokes 20 cigarettes per day and drinks 12 units of alcohol per week.

Examination

This man's jugular venous pressure (JVP) is not raised. Heart sounds are normal. The chest is clear to auscultation, with no evidence of peripheral oedema. Abdominal examination is normal. There is no lymphadenopathy, clubbing or skin rashes. Musculoskeletal examination is normal. An ECG (Fig. 88.1) shows less than 1 mm ST elevation in the inferior leads; PR interval normal; QRS normal duration and shape. Axis was normal. A chest X-ray shows mild cardiomegaly on a PA film. Lung fields are clear. Observations: temperature 37.8°C, heart rate 101/min, blood pressure 145/62 mmHg, respiratory rate 20/min, SaO_2 98 per cent on room air, blood sugar 5.2 mmol/L.

INVESTIGATIONS		
		Normal range
White cells	13.2	$4–11 \times 10^9$/L
Neutrophils	8.0	$2–7 \times 10^9$/L
Lymphocytes	2.7	$1–4.8 \times 10^9$/L
Haemoglobin	14.4	13–18 g/dL
Platelets	350	$150–400 \times 10^9$/L
Sodium	137	135–145 mmol/L
Potassium	4.2	3.5–5.0 mmol/L
Urea	4.0	3.0–7.0 mmol/L
Creatinine	68	60–110 µmol/L
C-reactive protein	154	<5 mg/L
Troponin-T	1.4	<0.03 µg/L
Arterial blood gas sample:		
pH	7.43	7.35–7.45
PO_2	7.4	9.3–13.3 kPa
PCO_2	3.1	4.7–6.0 kPa
Lactate	2.7	<2 mmol/L
HCO_3	24	22–26 mmol/L
Base excess:	+1	−3 to +3 mmol/L
Saturation	87%	>94%

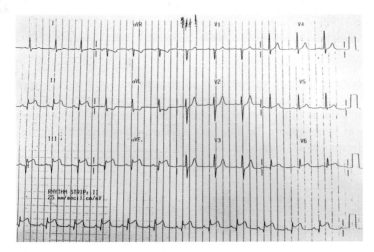

Figure 88.1

Questions
- What are the differential diagnoses?
- How would you further investigate this patient?

ANSWER 88

This man's ECG (Fig. 88.1) shows inferior changes with a raised troponin in keeping with myocardial damage. However, the aetiology is not immediately obvious. He presents with a fever and raised inflammatory markers with a prodromal illness. Apart from hypertension he has no risk factors for ischaemic heart disease. These symptoms fit best with myocarditis. Myocarditis is uncommon, but tends to affect young adults. Acute myocarditis can present mildly, as in this case, or in extremis with cardiogenic shock or sudden death. The causes of myocarditis include infections (viral being the most common – parvovirus B-19, adenovirus, coxsackie B, human herpes virus-6, cytomegalovirus, Epstein–Barr virus, herpes simplex, HIV), autoimmune diseases (e.g. systemic lupus erythematosus, rheumatoid arthritis) and drug-induced (anthracyclines).

He is haemodynamically stable and there is no evidence of heart failure. An echocardiogram will determine whether there is any left ventricular functional impairment and determine any regional wall motion abnormalities. He may well have inferior wall motion abnormalities as the ECG suggested some inferior changes. An echocardiogram will also identify an associated pericardial effusion. In view of the ST changes inferiorly on ECG and raised troponin, a coronary angiogram will need to be performed to ensure normal coronary anatomy. A sensitive and specific test to help confirm the diagnosis of myocarditis is an MRI with gadolinium enhancement. Typically parts of myocardium with late gadolinium enhancement identify areas of inflammation. The pattern of inflammation can help determine the type of myocarditis. Rarely endocardial biopsy is required to make the diagnosis or assist in management. Serological tests to identify viral causes would be indicated. If there is reason to suspect a connective tissue disease, other tests to identify the disorder can be performed.

Management in this case will be supportive. Monitoring for complications of myocarditis such as heart failure, conduction abnormalities or rarely tamponade from a pericardial effusion are required in the immediate term. Long-term complications include a dilated cardiomyopathy with chronic heart failure.

 KEY POINTS

- Myocarditis is uncommon but occurs in younger individuals and is most often due to a viral cause.
- Acute myocarditis can mimic an acute myocardial infarction and complications can include heart failure and conduction abnormalities.

CASE 89: DETERIORATING RENAL FUNCTION

History

A 73-year-old woman has been admitted with *Escherichia coli* bacteraemia secondary to pyelonephritis. Her history includes type 2 diabetes, hypertension, obesity and osteoarthritis. She is taking a multitude of drugs: metformin, 1 g twice daily; levemir, 16 units once daily; candesartan, 32 mg once daily; paracetamol, 1 g four times a day; spironolactone, 12.5 mg once daily; and atorvastatin, 10 mg once daily.

Initial treatment

Candesartan was stopped on admission owing to her low blood pressure. She received a seven-day course of gentamicin and had a good clinical response. The investigation results were obtained on admission and on day seven after admission.

INVESTIGATIONS		
		Normal range
On admission		
Sodium	137	135–145 mmol/L
Potassium	3.8	3.5–5.0 mmol/L
Urea	7	3.0–7.0 mmol/L
Creatinine	120	60–110 µmol/L
Urine dipstick	Blood 2+, protein negative, nitrites positive, leu 2+	
Day 7 after admission		
Sodium	140	135–145 mmol/L
Potassium	6.0	3.5–5.0 mmol/L
Urea	35	3.0–7.0 mmol/L
Creatinine	300	60–110 µmol/L
Urine dipstick:	Blood, protein, nitrites, leu all negative	

Questions

- What are the possible causes of her change in urea and electrolyte results?
- How would you manage this patient?

The blood results are highly suggestive of an acute kidney injury (AKI). This is defined by any functional, structural or markers of kidney damage occurring in the previous three months. AKI is one of a few classifications for acute renal failure – a historical term used to describe this condition.

AKI is divided into stages 1 to 3 and follows two criteria: (i) creatinine (Cr) and (ii) urine output (UO). Only one of the two criteria is needed for staging of AKI.

- Stage 1 = Cr increase >150–200% from baseline or UO <0.5 mL/kg/h for more than 6 hours.
- Stage 2 = Cr increase >200–300% from baseline or UO <0.5 mL/kg/h for more than 12 hours.
- Stage 3 = Cr increase >300% or Cr >350 μmol/L with acute rise of Cr >45 μmol/L or on renal replacement therapy or UO <0.3 mL/kg/h for 12 hours or anuria for 12 hours.

Mortality rate increases with more advanced stages of AKI.

The initial management of AKI is to look for the underlying cause(s) and to reverse the immediate life-threatening complication associated with AKI. The causes of AKI are classified into:

- prerenal (hypotension, hypovolaemia, renovascular disease);
- renal parenchymal (acute tubular necrosis, vasculitis, glomerular disorders or tubulo-interstitial disorders);
- postrenal (urine outflow obstruction).

While the aetiology is being investigated it is important to review the patient's intravascular volume status (i.e. intravascular fluid depletion or fluid overload) and potassium level. These are potentially lethal associated conditions that must be dealt with urgently.

The approach for any AKI patient should include the following.

- Look for a history of systemic disorders that may contribute to current AKI (e.g. vascular diseases, diabetes, rheumatological disorders, myeloma, sepsis).
- Examine volume status and decide whether volume replacement or diuresis is needed. Careful charting of fluid balance is important to monitor treatment response and to set therapeutic goals.
- Examine for palpable bladder/enlarged prostate and loin pain. It is important to insert a urinary catheter to exclude bladder outflow obstruction.
- Measure electrolytes and obtain an arterial/venous blood gas to review potassium and bicarbonate levels. Acidaemia often worsens hyperkalaemia and oral/intravenous sodium bicarbonate may sometimes be considered. A 12-lead ECG is needed to look for associated arrhythmia, especially when hyperkalaemia is present.
- Unless the patient is anuric, it is imperative to obtain a urine sample for dipstick, microbiology sampling and cytological assessment. 'Bland' urine dipstick (all negative results) is highly suggestive of prerenal AKI and acute tubular necrosis (ATN). Other rarer causes of bland urine are scleroderma, atherosclerotic emboli and tubulointerstitial disorders. Blood on dipstick may suggest glomerulonephritis, vasculitis, thrombotic microangiopathy, haemoglobinuria, myoglobinuria or trauma. Heavy proteinuria may be suggestive of nephrotic syndrome. Presence of white cells is suggestive of urinary tract infection or acute interstitial nephritis (eosinophils). Crystals found on urine examination may suggest urate nephropathy or drug-induced nephropathy (e.g.

ethylene glycol/acyclovir). Urinary sodium and osmolality can sometimes help differentiate prerenal AKI from ATN, but in practice it is often difficult due to concurrent diuretic therapy.

- Perform urgent ultrasound of the renal tract to exclude urinary tract obstruction, examine for asymmetrical kidney size secondary to ischaemic nephropathy and also to look for evidence of atrophic kidneys which is highly suggestive of advanced chronic kidney disease (an exception is diabetic nephropathy which retains 'normal' size kidneys).
- Look for evidence of chronic anaemia, hyperphosphataemia or hypocalcaemia which may suggest prior chronic kidney disease.
- Review recent drug histories carefully and stop all nephrotoxins. Also look for recent prescription of radiological contrast (weeks).
- In selected cases it may be important to request: liver function test (low albumin of nephrotic syndrome or hepatorenal syndrome); creatine kinase; urate (tumour lysis syndrome); lactate (hypoperfusion); prostate-specific antigen; antinuclear antibody; antineutrophil cytoplasmic antibody; rheumatoid factor; complement level; cryoglobulin level; hepatitis B and C serology; serum immunoglobulins; serum protein electrophoresis (myeloma). All systemic disorders may lead to kidney disease.

When to start, which modality to use and when to stop renal replacement therapy (haemodialysis or haemofiltration or both) are often debated. The emergency indications are (i) refractory or rapidly worsening hyperkalaemia, and (ii) diuresis-resistant acute pulmonary oedema. Other indications for dialysis are (a) intractable metabolic acidosis (pH <7.1), (b) uraemic pericarditis/encephalopathy, (c) poison removal (e.g. lithium), and (d) hyperthermia.

In the given scenario the two possible causes are acute tubular necrosis secondary to recent severe sepsis and/or gentamicin therapy. Gentamicin is an aminoglycoside antibiotic with a narrow therapeutic range. Aminoglycoside toxicity most commonly manifests as ototoxicity and nephrotoxicity which is dose-dependent. The risk is related to the trough concentration rather than the peak concentration, so careful daily serum concentration monitoring is important. Studies suggest once-daily dosing of gentamicin is associated with less nephrotoxicity without affecting its bactericidal efficacy, so it is the more commonly used regimen. Often aminoglycosides can cause renal failure and the accumulated level of drugs can further exacerbate this.

Gentamicin nephrotoxicity usually presents seven days after initiation of therapy. It may also occur even after therapy is stopped. In most cases it is reversible upon aminoglycoside withdrawal. Risk factors include severe intercurrent illness, history of chronic kidney disease, diabetes, use of iodine-based radiological contrast and concurrent use of potentially nephrotoxic drugs (e.g. non-steroidal anti-inflammatory drugs).

Gentamicin is dosed by *ideal* body weight (not actual body weight) and the daily maximum dose is 450 mg. A lower dose is often used in patients at risk of aminoglycoside nephropathy.

Other management considerations include stopping metformin as it is excreted unchanged in urine, and data suggest that Cr >150 μmol/L is the threshold for withholding metformin as it increases risk of lactic acidosis. Spironolactone is a potassium-sparing diuretic and is best avoided in AKI also.

KEY POINTS

- Be familiar with the investigation and treatment of acute kidney injury.
- Drugs can cause acute kidney injury, so a thorough drug history should be taken.
- The renal drug handling changes with alteration in renal function, so frequent reviews are needed to avoid toxicity.

History

A 67-year-old Caucasian man has presented to the emergency department complaining of flu-like symptoms and generalized weakness. He was well until six months ago, but since then he has had three episodes of pneumonia. Over the past week he developed dizziness, cough, diarrhoea, vomiting and progressive weakness. He was unable to get up from his bed on the day of presentation. His medical history includes ischaemic heart disease. He is an active smoker with 40 pack years history, but there is no history of alcohol or substance misuse. He has not travelled abroad in the last 10 years. He takes certain drugs: aspirin, 75 mg once daily; atenolol, 50 mg once daily; isosorbide mononitrate MR, 30 mg once daily.

Examination

This man looks unwell – dehydrated with dry lips and reduced skin turgor. Postural hypotension is noted. His jugular venous pulse (JVP) is not visible in the recumbent position. Heart sounds are normal. Chest examination reveals right lower zone crackles with bronchial breathing in the same area on auscultation, but a chest X-ray shows clear lung fields. An ECG reveals sinus tachycardia. Observations: temperature 36.5°C, heart rate 120/min, blood pressure 100/60 mmHg, respiratory rate 28/min, SaO_2 92 per cent on room air.

INVESTIGATIONS		
		Normal range
White cells	5.0	4–11×10^9/L
Neutrophils	2.8	2–7×10^9/L
Haemoglobin	10.0	13–18 g/dL
Platelets	168	150–400×10^9/L
Sodium	115	135–145 mmol/L
Potassium	6.0	3.5–5.0 mmol/L
Urea	10	3.0–7.0 mmol/L
Creatinine	100	60–110 µmol/L
C-reactive protein	70	<5 mg/L
Blood gas sample on room air:		
pH	7.31	7.35–7.45
PO_2	8.0	9.3–13.3 kPa
PCO_2	3.0	4.7–6.0 kPa
Lactate	3.0	<2 mmol/L
HCO_3	18	22–26 mmol/L
Base excess	−4	−3 to +3 mmol/L

Questions

- What is the unifying diagnosis of this man's presentation?
- How would you manage this patient in an acute general medical setting?

ANSWER 90

This man is clearly very unwell. His blood tests show a dangerously low sodium, a high potassium and a probable acute kidney injury. His C-reactive protein is also elevated, showing that there is likely to be a degree of underlying inflammation or infection. The arterial blood gas sample is consistent with a lactic acidosis with a compensatory respiratory alkalosis. All of these findings are reflective of his critical illness. The suspicion is that he has Addison's disease.

This man should be nursed and fully monitored in a high-dependency area. His breathing should be supported with high-flow oxygen to target an oxygen saturation of at least 94 per cent. Multiple large-bore intravenous accesses should be established as soon as possible for the treatment of hypoglycaemia and dehydration. A urinary catheter should be inserted to record urine output, and this will give a rough indication of renal perfusion and renal function, which in turn can guide intravenous fluid therapy. A bolus of fluid should be given as fluid challenge as soon as possible. It is important to re-examine this man frequently to review his fluid status so that fluid therapy can be targeted correctly without causing fluid overload. This is particularly important in patients with a history of ischaemic heart disease or heart failure. Repeat blood samples (arterial or venous) should be taken to track changes in sodium, potassium, lactate, glucose and metabolic acidosis. Plasma sodium level should be not be raised more rapidly than a rate of 1–2 mmol per hour up to a level of 125 mmol/L to prevent central pontine myelinolysis. Antibiotics for the treatment of community-acquired pneumonia should be initiated without delay. As this man had a previous chest infection, it may be important to look for previous laboratory sputum or blood cultures and to target antibiotic therapy accordingly.

Dehydration, hyponatraemia, hyperkalaemia, metabolic acidosis, hypoglycaemia and hypercalcaemia are features of hypoadrenal crisis. The immediate management plan should aim to support blood glucose, restore fluid and electrolyte imbalance and to replace steroids. Although it is important to obtain a 9 am plasma ACTH (adrenocorticotropic hormone) and cortisol level and to perform a short ACTH stimulation test to diagnose adrenal insufficiency, patients are often too unwell and these tests should not delay the administration of fluid and steroids (e.g. hydrocortisone). A random sample of cortisol should ideally be taken before steroid therapy. High-dose steroid treatment in hypoadrenal crisis has sufficient mineralocorticoid activity and fludrocortisone can be introduced later.

With regard to the differential diagnosis of hyponatraemia in this scenario, it would be impossible to diagnose syndrome of inappropriate antidiuretic hormone (ADH) secretion as he is clinically dehydrated. A spot urinary sodium sample at initial presentation is sometimes helpful as urinary Na above 20 mmol/L in a dehydrated patient with hyponatraemia without diuretic therapy should raise suspicion of adrenal insufficiency.

KEY POINTS

- The presenting symptoms of Addison's disease are non-specific, so a high index of suspicion is needed to make the diagnosis.
- It is ideal to take 9 am cortisol blood sample and perform a Synacthen® test to make the diagnosis of Addison's disease prior to instigating steroid treatment. However, in an acute medical emergency, empirical steroid should be given without delay.

CASE 91: BLURRED VISION WITH HEADACHE

History

A 32-year-old Caucasian man has presented to the emergency eye clinic with blurred vision. It has worsened over the past two days and has been accompanied by severe headache for a week. He has also been suffering from frequent intermittent headaches over the past year. These are generalized and tend to occur at any time through the day, with no association with eye symptoms until now. He has no history of epilepsy, muscle weakness, dizziness, hearing loss or weight loss. His blurred vision is worst in the left eye.

Examination

This man looks well. His cardiorespiratory and abdominal examinations are unremarkable. Examination of the eyes reveals intact visual fields and eye movements. Visual acuity is 6/6 in the right eye and 6/24 in the left. There is enlargement of the blind spot. Direct ophthalmoscopy shows bilateral papilloedema. There is a cotton-wool spot over the left macula and multiple flame haemorrhages. There are no other cranial or peripheral nervous system defects. His blood pressure is persistently 260/140 mmHg, measured sitting.

INVESTIGATIONS		
		Normal range
White cells	6.0	$4-11 \times 10^9/L$
Haemoglobin	14.0	13–18 g/dL
Platelets	200	$150-400 \times 10^9/L$
Sodium	137	135–145 mmol/L
Potassium	3.7	3.5–5.0 mmol/L
Urea	12	3.0–7.0 mmol/L
Creatinine	144	60–110 µmol/L

Question

• How would you manage this patient acutely?

The definition of severe hypertension varies, but most clinicians would agree a figure of >180/110 mmHg. When faced with a very high blood pressure the first step is to decide, through clinical assessment, whether a patient is in 'hypertensive urgency' or 'hypertensive emergency'.

Assessment of severe hypertension should be targeted towards investigation of target organ damage. These are hypertensive encephalopathy, stroke, acute left ventricular failure, acute coronary syndrome, aortic dissection and renal impairment.

- Hypertensive urgency is characterized by severe hypertension without acute target organ damage.
- Hypertensive emergency is characterized by severe hypertension with acute target damage as listed above.

Assessment of target organ damage begins with history-taking for symptoms suggesting ischaemic heart disease, heart failure, peripheral vascular disease, or cerebrovascular disease. Examinations should include clinical signs of heart failure, peripheral vascular examinations including auscultation of carotid and renal bruit, and examining for radio-femoral pulse delay, palpable kidneys, lateralizing neurological signs and direct fundoscopy to look for papilloedema. Also evaluate for evidence of obstructive sleep apnoea as it is often associated with refractory hypertension (treatment of this condition can enhance long-term blood pressure lowering).

Investigate global cardiovascular risk and possible secondary causes of severe hypertension, such as primary hyperaldosteronism, phaeochromocytoma, renovascular hypertension, or coarctation of the aorta. This should include urine samples (proteinuria and haematuria and 24-hour urinary catecholamine levels), and blood samples (for potassium, creatinine, fasting blood glucose and lipid profile and renin and aldosterone levels). Perform an ECG to look for evidence of left ventricular hypertrophy, arrhythmias or previous myocardial infarction.

Hypertensive encephalopathy occurs when the brain loses its ability to autoregulate its own perfusion in the context of severe hypertension. It leads to cerebral oedema and manifests with symptoms and signs of headache, nausea and vomiting, papilloedema, and sometimes lateralizing neurological signs. Hypertensive encephalopathy is a diagnosis of exclusion, so neuroimaging should be requested urgently to exclude stroke, encephalitis or an intracranial space-occupying lesion. When this diagnosis is suspected, the patient should be nursed in a high-dependency area. An arterial line should be inserted to allow continuous blood pressure measurements.

Hypertensive urgency should be treated mainly with oral antihypertensive therapy as per local guidelines. The aim is to lower the mean arterial pressure (MAP) no more than 25 per cent of the presenting MAP or in the region of 160/110 mmHg over 24–72 hours. Patients should be evaluated every 72 hours. From previous experience of blood pressure trials, it is likely that a second or even third antihypertensive agent is needed to achieve effective blood pressure control, and this should be considered early. If an angiotensin-converting enzyme (ACE) inhibitor, angiotensin receptor blocker (ARB) or diuretic is prescribed, close monitoring of renal function and potassium is very important. Oral nifedipine MR (modified release; not sublingual) is a safe agent to start with. Amlodipine is often used but it takes a week to exert its full pharmacological effect, so nifedipine MR is preferable. This can be switched over to amlodipine once blood pressure is stabilized.

Patients likely to have low renin hypertension (black patients of any age, or any patient aged >55) are more likely to respond to diuretic therapy. In resistant hypertension it is not uncommon to use a thiazide or loop diuretic with a potassium-sparing diuretic for the treatment of hypertension.

Despite the name, intravenous antihypertensive treatment is not always necessarily needed for a hypertensive emergency. The general goal is to reduce the MAP no more than 25 per cent over 4 hours and to aim for blood pressure in the region of 160/110 mmHg in 24 hours. Situations that need intravenous treatment include hypertensive encephalopathy, aortic dissection, acute coronary syndrome and acute left ventricular failure. Intravenous antihypertensives can reduce blood pressure very quickly (in minutes), so close monitoring is necessary to avoid abrupt reductions in brain, kidney and coronary perfusion. Intravenous glyceryl trinitrate, sodium nitroprusside, hydralazine, labetolol and phentolamine are intravenous agents often used in this situation. Conventional beta-blockers such as bisoprolol and metoprolol are ineffective as single agents in hypertensive emergencies, presumably due to the lack of vasodilating properties. However, in aortic dissection and arrhythmia conventional beta-blockers should be added.

 KEY POINTS

- Severe hypertension is diagnosed when the blood pressure exceeds 180/110 mmHg.
- The aim should be to lower the mean arterial pressure by no more than 25 per cent of the presenting MAP, so oral agents may be preferable to intravenous agents.

History
A 69-year-old woman has presented to the emergency department with a two-day history of severe right upper quadrant abdominal pain. This was colicky in nature initially but has now progressed to constant abdominal pain. Her pain is associated with dark urine, and her children noticed she had yellow discolouration on her skin and her eye in the morning when they came to visit her. She also reports poor oral intake over the past week and has felt feverish with rigor since yesterday. She was previously fit and well.

Examination
This woman is icteric and looks unwell with reduced skin turgor and dry tongue. She feels cool to the touch up to her wrists and her ankles. There is no clubbing or lymphadenopathy. Her jugular venous pulse (JVP) cannot be seen and her pulse volume is reduced. Capillary refill is 2 seconds. The cardiorespiratory examination is otherwise normal. There is tenderness in the upper abdomen with positive Murphy's sign. Bowel sounds are present. A rectal examination is unremarkable. Observations: temperature 39°C, heart rate 120/min, blood pressure 98/57 mmHg, respiratory rate 28/min, SaO_2 93 per cent on room air.

INVESTIGATIONS		
		Normal range
White cells	20.0	$4–11 \times 10^9$/L
Neutrophils	18.4	$2–7 \times 10^9$/L
Haemoglobin	12.8	13–18 g/dL
Platelets	180	$150–400 \times 10^9$/L
Sodium	135	135–145 mmol/L
Potassium	3.6	3.5–5.0 mmol/L
Urea	12	3.0–7.0 mmol/L
Creatinine	180	60–110 µmol/L
C-reactive protein	310	<5 mg/L
Amylase	300	20–110 IU/L
Bilirubin	80	5–25 µmol/L
Alanine aminotransferase	100	8–55 IU/L
Alkaline phosphatase	340	42–98 IU/L
Albumin	30	35–50 g/L
Gamma-glytamyl transpeptidase	111	8–78 IU/L
INR	1.8	0.9–1.1
Arterial blood gas on room air:		
pH	7.29	7.35–7.45
PO_2	11.0	9.3–13.3 kPa
PCO_2	3.2	4.7–6.0 kPa
Lactate	4.0	<2 mmol/L
HCO_3	18	22–26 mmol/L
Base excess	−4	−3 to +3 mmol/L

Questions
- What is the most likely diagnosis?
- How would you manage this woman?

Fever, jaundice and right upper quadrant abdominal pain make up the Charcot's triad which are the main signs and symptoms of acute cholangitis. If a patient presents with Charcot's triad and altered mental status and shock, it is called Reynold's pentad. This woman has presented with Reynold's pentad and will require urgent resuscitation.

The most common cause of acute cholangitis is gallstone disease. Other causes are tumours (such as pancreatic cancer or cholangiocarcinoma) and strictures associated with previous biliary tree instrumentation. These processes lead to biliary tract outflow obstruction and bacterial infection. The most common bacteria are Gram-negative organisms such as *Escherichia coli*, although Enterococci and anaerobes could also be responsible.

The first step of this patient's resuscitation is to ensure she is fully monitored in a high-dependency area. Oxygen should be given to ensure SaO_2 of at least 94 per cent. Intravenous access and blood cultures should be taken, and intravenous fluid and antibiotics should be given as soon as possible. A colloid bolus fluid challenge should be delivered to ensure her mean arterial pressure (MAP) is above 65 mmHg. Mean arterial pressure is used as the resuscitation target as it is more closely related to organ perfusion. This woman has evidence of acute kidney injury, so a urinary catheter should be inserted to monitor urine output. Reviewing clinical status frequently is very important in the resuscitation of any critically ill patient.

Part of the Surviving Sepsis guidelines (http://www.survivingsepsis.org) highlight the importance of 'source identification and control'. As acute cholangitis is caused by biliary obstruction it is important to establish what is causing the blockage. An urgent ultrasound of the abdomen should be arranged to look for gallstones and a dilated common bile duct. In experienced hands, ultrasound of the biliary tree is the best modality in identifying gallstones. Another increasingly common modality to be used is magnetic resonance cholangiopancreatography (MRCP), which gives a clear image of the anatomy of the biliary tree and the pancreatic duct. Therapeutic endoscopic retrograde cholangiopancreatography (ERCP) is useful in relieving obstructing gallstones in the common bile duct, and to insert stent(s) for malignant strictures to temporarily relieve biliary obstruction.

 KEY POINTS

- Acute cholangitis carries a high mortality.
- It is important to treat acute cholangitis promptly with antibiotics and control the source as appropriate.

History

An unkempt man has been brought to the emergency department, having been found collapsed in the street. Earlier he was seen sitting in the street confused and agitated. An empty two-litre cider bottle was found in his possession. He is unable to give a history.

Initial treatment

Shortly after arrival he started having a generalized seizure which self-terminated in 3 minutes. Supplemental oxygen was given and intravenous access was established. His Glasgow Coma Scale score after the seizure was 4/15 (E1, V2, M1). While the attending doctor was assessing this man he began to have another generalized seizure. A dose of lorazepam 4 mg was given intravenously and was repeated after 10 minutes as he continued to have seizures.

🔍 INVESTIGATIONS

Arterial blood gas sample

	15 L oxygen	Normal range
pH	7.25	7.35–7.45
PO_2	25	9.3–13.3 kPa
PCO_2	3.2	4.7–6.0 kPa
Lactate	4.0	<2 mmol/L
HCO_3	19	22–26 mmol/L
Base excess	−8	−3 to +3 mmol/L

Question

• What should be the immediate management plan for this patient?

The immediate management should consist of the following.

A   Maintain a patent airway by laying this man in the recovery position. If possible: chin lift, controlled suction, oropharyngeal airway if appropriate.
B   Apply high-flow oxygen and assess respiratory rate and targeted chest assessment.
C   Monitor heart rate and blood pressure, and fluid resuscitate as appropriate.
D   Glucose is very important in any patient presenting with seizure and should be assessed immediately. Assess for focal neurological signs suggesting a focal brain lesion.

Any sick patient should be monitored in a high-dependency area. A useful acronym is MOVE:

M   Monitoring (cardiorespiratory);
O   give Oxygen;
V   establish Venous access;
E   perform 12-lead ECG.

An arterial blood gas is always a useful test when a patient is unwell. The blood gas results of this patient show that the patient has an acidosis (pH <7.35). The patient is well oxygenated (on 15 L of O_2 via a non-rebreathing mask), and his PCO_2 is slightly lower than normal, so this is not a respiratory acidosis. His bicarbonate level is low and his lactate level is high. This is a metabolic acidosis, which has probably resulted from earlier tissue hypoxia.

The National Institute for Health and Clinical Excellence guideline CG20 (Epilepsy in adults and children, 2004) consists of a useful protocol for the management of acute seizure and status epilepticus. All practitioners of acute medicine should be familiar with the protocol.

Once a seizure is identified, always shout for help because it is impossible to execute ABC + MOVE on your own. Look at your watch and note the time because it is useful in deciding what to do next.

Status epilepticus is defined as a seizure lasting more than 30 minutes, or a patient having repeat seizures without regaining consciousness for over 30 minutes. Although the timeline on a conventional seizure treatment algorithm is very helpful, it is important to 'anticipate' rather than waiting for the next timepoint on the guideline to act (e.g. it takes time to draw up a lorazepam and phentyoin infusion). The timepoints serve as a guide only; in some circumstances it will be appropriate to expediate or delay a treatment according to the clinical situation. In this patient, intravenous dextrose and thiamine should be given as there is a suspicion of alochol-related seizure. Try to look for clues for seizure; for example, look for signs of head trauma (subdural or extradural haematoma), stroke, poisoning (methanol, ethylene glycol, paracetamol, etc.), or infection (encephalitis, meningitis). Correct hypotension and metabolic abnormalities as swiftly as possible.

Lorazepam is the preferred benzodiazepine in the United Kingdom as the first-line treatment of acute seizure. Lorazepam reaches a peak plasma concentration after 5 minutes, with peak central nervous system (CNS) effects by 30 minutes. Although intravenous diazepam is more rapid in onset of action, the significantly longer duration of action of lorazepam makes it a preferable drug as it is effective for up to 5–8 hours. Diazepam has a shorter duration in the CNS as it rapidly distributes in fat and tissues. Lorazepam should be given in a bolus at a maximum dose of 4 mg, and this can be repeated once in 10–20 minutes if seizures are not terminated. In instances where intravenous access is not possible, rectal diazepam 10 mg should be given. Peak concentration is reached in 10–20 minutes when diazepam is given rectally. If the seizure is terminated and the patient is able to swallow safely, they should be given their usual antiepileptic if they are known to have a diagnosis of epilepsy.

Intravenous phenytoin should be prepared as soon as possible when a repeated dose of benzodiazepine is given, as in the patient described. At this point the status epilepticus is established and anaesthetists and the intensive-care team should be alerted. Give phenytoin (15 mg/kg at a rate of 50 mg/min) as soon as it is feasible if the seizure is continuing. In refractory status epilepticus, a general anaesthetic drug such as thiopentone or propofol is often used. All agents used in the treatment of acute seizure have significant negative inotropic effects, so close cardiovascular monitoring is needed. Phenytoin is itself a class Ib Vaughan–Williams antiarrhythmic and, although its use in arrhythmia is obsolete, it acts on the cardiac sodium channel and shortens action potential, therefore ECG monitoring is needed. Cardiac patients especially with conduction abnormalities should be given phenytoin with caution. Phenytoin should be given into a large vein if possible as it is very alkaline and may cause phlebitis: this can be quite severe and cause a 'purple glove syndrome'. Phenytoin should be diluted with normal saline as dextrose solution causes precipitation. Blood sugar should be monitored regularly as phenytoin can potentially cause both hyper- and hypoglycaemia.

When seizures are under control, consider neuroimaging to identify the underlying cause of presentation. All patients with a first seizure should receive follow-up and driving advice.

 KEY POINT

- The treatment algorithm of generalized seizure and status epilepticus is important to learn as it is a common medical emergency.

History

An 82-year-old man presented with a three-day history of watery diarrhoea and fever. This was associated with worsening left-sided abdominal pain which started yesterday. It was described as constant and sharp, and not relieved by defecation. This diarrhoea occurred up to ten times per day and was not associated with rectal bleeding. There was no recent travel history and he had been cooking all his meals. His medical history includes hypertension and he takes amlodipine 5 mg once daily.

Examination

This man showed no lymphadenopathy. Cardiorespiratory and neurological examinations were unremarkable. The abdomen was tender in the left iliac fossa with guarding and hyperactive bowel sounds. Observations: temperature 38.0°C, heart rate 100/min, blood pressure 110/55 mmHg, respiratory rate 20/min, SaO_2 97 per cent on room air.

Initial treatment

He was admitted for intravenous antibiotics for presumptive diverticulitis. Twelve hours later he complains of worsening abdominal pain and new-onset left thigh pain. His abdomen is rigid with absent bowel sounds. His left iliac fossa and left thigh are very tender, with an extensive erythematous rash covering the left thigh from the knee up to the groin. New observations: temperature 39°C, heart rate 120/min, blood pressure 98/55 mmHg, respiratory rate 24/min, SaO_2 97 per cent on room air.

INVESTIGATIONS		
		Normal range
White cells	32.0	$4–11 \times 10^9$/L
Haemoglobin	13.0	13–18 g/dL
Platelets	140	$150–400 \times 10^9$/L
Sodium	130	135–145 mmol/L
Potassium	2.8	3.5–5.0 mmol/L
Urea	12	3.0–7.0 mmol/L
Creatinine	120	60–110 µmol/L
C-reactive protein	458	<5 mg/L
INR	1.8	0.9–1.1
Arterial blood gas on room air:		
pH	7.37	7.35–7.45
PO_2	10.0	9.3–13.3 kPa
PCO_2	3.2	4.7–6.0 kPa
Lactate	6.0	<2 mmol/L
HCO_3	18	22–26 mmol/L
Base excess	−8	−3 to +3 mmol/L

Questions

- What is the most likely diagnosis?
- How would you manage this condition?

This man presented with diverticulitis and one of the known complications is perforation. The finding of a new, tender, erythematous rash is worrying as infected material from perforated bowel could potentially spread to surrounding soft tissues, leading to necrotizing fasciitis.

The immediate management requires rapid stabilization of septic shock using goal-directed therapy according to the Surviving Sepsis guidelines (http://www.surviving sepsis.org). The rapidly progressing nature of necrotizing fasciitis necessitates urgent surgical intervention for source control or debridement of necrotic tissue and resection of the affected bowel.

Necrotizing fasciitis is a rapidly fatal condition affecting the skin. The offending organism(s) spread through the fascial compartments and release toxins. This leads to infective vasculitis and thrombus formation, resulting in vascular occlusion and tissue necrosis. This corresponds to a clinical finding of painful erythematous rash (sometimes bullus formation) which may progress to gangrenous discolouration if untreated. Crepitation is a classical finding but may not be present unless a gas-forming organism is involved.

Necrotizing fasciitis can be divided into different types according to the microbiological agent(s) involved:

- type 1 (polymicrobial);
- type 2 (group A *Streptococcus*);
- type 3 (*Clostridia* – known to cause gas gangerene).

Mortality can approach 70 per cent. Prompt surgical debridement is the key and antibiotics alone are insufficient to alter the course of this illness.

In this case, the diagnosis of necrotizing fasciitis was made and the man went to theatre for debridement of the infected tissue. Despite the surgical intervention the infection progressed and he developed a large deep vein thrombosis in his left leg. He ultimately required a left above-knee amputation. After intensive physiotherapy and assistance from the occupational therapists, he made a good recovery.

 KEY POINTS

- Necrotizing fasciitis is a rapidly progressive and life-threatening condition affecting the skin and underlying tissues.
- Surgical debridement plus antibiotic and fluid management will be necessary in order to remove any infected tissue.

History
A 19-year-old man has presented to his GP with a one-day history of rapid onset of multiple target-like skin lesions. This is associated with sore throat, mouth and lips, and red eyes. He also complains of fever and malaise preceding the onset of the skin lesions. He is fit, with no previous history of any skin disorder or allergy. Seven days earlier he twisted his ankle while playing football and had taken paracetamol and ibuprofen for a few days.

Examination
This young man looks unwell. He has conjunctival injection bilaterally. There are multiple irregular erosions in the mouth and on the lips that are tender with haemorrhagic crusting. There are widespread erythematous lesions over all four limbs. Observations: temperature 37.9°C, heart rate 120/min, blood pressure 80/50 mmHg, respiratory rate 24/min, SaO_2 99 per cent on room air.

INVESTIGATIONS		
		Normal range
Arterial blood gas on room air:		
pH	7.37	7.35–7.45
PO_2	12	9.3–13.3 kPa
PCO_2	3.9	4.7–6.0 kPa
Lactate	4.3	<2 mmol/L
HCO_3	22	22–26 mmol/L
Base excess	−3	−3 to +3 mmol/L

Questions
- What are the differential diagnoses?
- How would you manage this young man?

ANSWER 95

The presence of extensive target-like lesions is highly suggestive of erythema multiforme major (EM major) or Stevens–Johnson syndrome (SJS). Some authorities suggest that EM, SJS and toxic epidermal necrolysis (TEN) have similar pathophysiological processes and differ only in the extent of dermatological and mucosal involvement. One classification suggests that EM minor is skin lesions without mucosal involvement. EM major or SJS is a more severe form of EM minor involving mucosal lesions. The extent of skin lesion in SJS is usually less than 10 per cent of the body surface area. TEN is a severe form of SJS where over 30 per cent body surface area is affected. In TEN, the dermis separates from the epidermis, causing extensive erosion and blisters (leading to a positive Nikolsky sign). The oral, conjunctival, respiratory, gastrointestinal and urogenital mucosae are also involved, leading to lip adhesion, corneal erosions, respiratory failure, upper gastrointestinal bleeding, urinary retention, sepsis and multi-organ failure. Scoring systems such as SCORTEN are available to predict TEN prognosis. Clinically it may be difficult to separate TEN and SJS as it may overlap.

Fifty per cent of cases of EM minor are idiopathic, and if an identifiable cause is found then it is due to one of the following categories: infection (e.g. herpes simplex, human immunodeficiency virus, mycoplasma, group A *Streptococcus*, malaria), a connective tissue disorder (e.g. systemic lupus erythematosus, vasculitides), malignancy (e.g. lymphoma) or drug-related (e.g. vaccination, antibiotic, anticonvulsant, non-steroidal anti-inflammatory drug). The causes of SJS and TEN are the same as for EM minor, although drugs are more likely to be implicated. The time between drug exposure and symptoms can vary between 4 and 28 days.

This patient is tachycardic and hypotensive. He needs prompt treatment with intravenous fluids. He may require antibiotics for a superadded bacterial infection from his skin lesions. If there is an on-call dermatologist available, he/she should be notified about the patient as soon as possible. These patients often become very unwell and require treatment in a high-dependency unit. You should notify the team there if the patient's blood pressure and heart rate do not improve after fluid resuscitation.

In EM minor, the rash settles in 2–3 weeks and the treatment is conservative. In SJS and TEN, the use of systemic steroids and intravenous immunoglobulin G are well documented in the literature but the results remain controversial. Supportive care in intensive care or a specialist unit is fundamental to the management of this condition. The general management is similar to that of erythroderma with special attention to good oral, skin and eye care. Instigate cardiorespiratory support as appropriate. Provide nutritional supplementation. Identification and prompt treatment of complications such as sepsis, good body temperature control and symptomatic relief are all important aspects of management of SJS and TEN. Stop all offending drugs and minimize unnecessary prescriptions.

With any severe adverse reaction to a drug (or any adverse reaction to a new drug) it is important to report the matter to the Medicines and Healthcare Products Agency (MHPA) through the yellow card scheme.

KEY POINTS

- The presence of target-like lesions in the context of a drug reaction is highly suggestive of erythema multiforme.
- As with erythroderma, it is important to recognize that this condition is a dermatological emergency that needs to be treated promptly.
- Withdraw all implicated drug therapy as soon as possible.

History

A 35-year-old woman has presented to the emergency department with fever, malaise and neck stiffness. She complains also of a vague history of headache, vertigo and insomnia over the past week. Today she developed fever, photophobia and neck stiffness and a red rash that is blanching and not purpuric. There is no personal history of dental or sinus diseases and no relevant drug history or travel history.

Examination

There is a symmetrical maculopapular rash involving this woman's entire body. In the perineum there are warty, plaque-like lesions. There are painless lymph nodes in the cervical, axillary and groin areas. There are no peripheral stigmata of subacute endocarditis. Her cardiorespiratory and abdominal examinations are unremarkable. Examination of the nervous system reveals mild neck stiffness, but the rest of the cranial nerves and peripheral nervous system examinations are unremarkable. Ophthalmoscopy reveals no abnormalities. A chest X-ray is normal. CT of the brain with intravenous contrast shows the presence of meningeal enhancement but no evidence of a space-occupying lesion. Observations: temperature 39.2°C, heart rate 110/min, blood pressure 110/70 mmHg, SaO_2 99 per cent on room air.

INVESTIGATIONS		
		Normal range
White cells	19.0	$4-11 \times 10^9$/L
Neutrophils	18	$2-7 \times 10^9$/L
Haemoglobin	13.0	13–18 g/dL
Platelets	244	$150-400 \times 10^9$/L
Sodium	136	135–145 mmol/L
Potassium	4.2	3.5–5.0 mmol/L
Urea	7.5	3.0–7.0 mmol/L
Creatinine	88	60–110 µmol/L
C-reactive protein	122	<5 mg/L
TPHA/treponemal antibody	Positive	

Lumbar puncture:
Opening pressure 20 mmHg (normal range 10–20)
CSF microscopy: predominately lymphocytes, 445/mm^3
Protein 1.2 g/L (normal range 0.2–0.4)
CSF culture negative
Cryptococcal antigen negative
Presence of reactive *Treponema pallidum* particle agglutination (TPPA) and Venereal Disease Research Laboratory (VDRL) test positive

Questions
- What is the appropriate initial management for this patient?
- What are the differential diagnoses?

ANSWER 96

This woman presented with meningitis and her initial management steps should be directed towards establishing the diagnosis rapidly and the administration of appropriate antibiotics without any delay. Blood cultures should be taken. A lumbar puncture has been performed. Contraindications for this are the presence of focal neurological signs such as limb weakness and brainstem signs, and/or papilloedema and/or depressed Glasgow Coma Scale score, especially <11, and/or seizures. Note that a 'normal' CT of brain in acute meningitis does not mean that lumbar puncture is completely safe. Clinical signs remain important pointers to risk stratification prior to performing a lumbar puncture. In suspected cases of meningococcal septicaemia, lumbar puncture is not needed and administration of antibiotics should be the priority.

In this case the cerebrospinal fluid (CSF) results showed lymphocytosis with elevated protein and low glucose compared to a paired serum sample. Common causes of this picture are tuberculous meningitis and fungal meningitis. Empirical antituberculous or antifungal treatment should be considered. In cases of pneumococcal and tuberculous meningitis, steroid therapy should be added for prognostic benefit. Viral meningitis would also lead to CSF lymphocytosis, but the rest of biochemistry is typically normal and this can be confirmed by appropriate virology tests. In older patients, *Listeria* meningitis can also lead to CSF lymphocytosis.

The presence of a generalized maculopapular rash and rashes suggestive of condylomata lata are typical of syphilis. The findings of positive reagin tests both in the serum and in the CSF support the diagnosis of acute syphilitic meningitis – a form of neurosyphilis. When syphilis is suspected it is important to consider HIV testing as these conditions often co-exist and syphilis enhances transmission of HIV. Contact tracing should be considered once syphilis or HIV is confirmed, and appropriate help should be sought from a sexual health clinic.

There are studies suggesting a resurgence of neurosyphilis in the era of HIV infection. It is thought that at least 30 per cent of cases of *Treponema pallidum* infection invade the central nervous system within days. Most patients (80 per cent) clear CNS *Treponema* infections without any clinical manifestations, but the rest are thought to present as acute early meningeal syphilis.

Treatment with penicillin arrests further well-known latent complications such as meningovascular syphilis, spinal syphilis, CNS gumma, generalized paresis of the insane, optic syphilis and tabes dorsalis. After a course of penicillin treatment, a CSF sample is repeated at six-month intervals until normal to monitor for treatment failure. This is especially important in HIV co-infection.

 KEY POINTS

- Neurosyphilis is a rare neurological disorder caused by *Treponema pallidum*.
- All patients diagnosed with a sexually transmitted disease should be offered HIV testing, as co-infection is common.

CASE 97: SEIZURE

History
A 62-year-old woman presented with inferior ST-elevation myocardial infarction. She was thrombolysed with tenectaplase and she remained well for 72 hours. On the fourth day after admission she had a grand mal seizure that self-terminated in 3 minutes. After the fit she remained drowsy. She is known to have ischaemic heart disease and hypertension. Her current medications are: aspirin, 75 mg once daily; ramipril, 2.5 mg once daily; bisoprolol, 5 mg once daily; atorvastatin, 40 mg once daily; GTN spray p.r.n.

Examination
On examination it appears that she is snoring, however her cardiorespiratory examination is otherwise normal. Her Glasgow Coma Scale score is 6/15 (E2, V1, M3). Pupils are equal and reactive to light bilaterally and there are spontaneous eye movements. There is no neck stiffness. The tone in all limbs is slightly raised. Reflexes are reduced globally. Bilateral clonus is present and both plantar responses are extensor. Observations: temperature 37.2°C, heart rate 120/min, blood pressure 150/90 mmHg, respiratory rate 28/min, SaO_2 92 per cent on room air.

INVESTIGATIONS		
		Normal range
Arterial blood gas on room air:		
pH	7.36	7.35–7.45
PO_2	8.2	9.3–13.3 kPa
PCO_2	5.2	4.7–6.0 kPa
Lactate	2.0	<2 mmol/L
HCO_3	23	22–26 mmol/L
Base excess	−2	−3 to +3 mmol/L

Questions
- What is the immediate concern with this patient?
- How would you further investigate this woman's current problem?

This woman had a recent myocardial infarction (MI) treated with thrombolytics. She had a self-terminating seizure and her consciousness level was depressed. An immediate concern is her snoring, which is indicative of partial upper airway obstruction. She should have an airway adjunct (e.g. oropharyngeal airway) inserted immediately and supplemental high-flow oxygen applied to bring up her oxygen saturation. She should be nursed in the recovery position for now.

It is important to check her blood sugar as it is a rapidly reversible cause of a seizure. More importantly, reassess airway, breathing and circulation until the patient is stabilized. She should be moved to a high-dependency area in the ward so that close monitoring is possible. Venous access should be established and blood taken to look for reversible causes of seizure such as electrolyte disturbances. Always perform a 12-lead ECG when feasible because 'seizure-like' activity (especially unwitnessed) could be caused by underlying cardiac arrhythmia (e.g. prolonged QT-interval syndrome could present as a morning tonic–clonic seizure). In addition, seizures can trigger cardiac arrhythmias.

Given the history of cardiovascular disease with target-organ damage (recent MI) and use of thrombolysis, the most important diagnosis to exclude here is a stroke. The presence of cardiovascular disease increases the probability of cerebrovascular pathology, or the mechanism might be a bleed related to the thrombolysis or embolus from thrombus in the left ventricle over an infarcted area. The incidence of stroke after thrombolysis is around 1–1.5 per cent and most strokes occur within five days of the MI, with most cases of haemorrhage within 24 hours of MI and thrombolysis. The given collection of neurological signs is not 'classical' for a stroke, and it is not possible to determine which circulation (anterior versus posterior arterial territories) is affected. However, most of the findings could be explained by a recent seizure. Findings of decorticate response (flexor response) to external stimuli and seizure in the context of a stroke suggest a large lesion above the brainstem. With this level of GCS score and impending airway obstruction, an urgent anaesthetic assessment should be sought with a view to intubation.

Once she is stable she should have urgent neuroimaging (CT or MRI) to look for evidence of intracerebral haemorrhage. The key to management of any post-stroke patient is attention to:

- reversal of vascular risk factors – anticoagulation for atrial fibrillation and antiplatelet therapy after ischaemic stroke, good blood pressure control, cholesterol and glucose control, internal carotid endarterectomy if indicated;
- nutritional support;
- focused neurorehabilitation from a stroke unit with multidisciplinary support – swallowing assessment, pressure sore prevention, temperature monitoring, deep vein thrombosis prophylaxis, speech and language therapy, physio- and occupational therapy.

In cases of intracerebral haemorrhage, anticoagulants and antiplatelets are contraindicated and long-term blood pressure control is very important. Neurosurgery has little role except in cases where haemorrhages are limited to the posterior fossa.

Thrombolysis is a new treatment modality for strokes and its use in the treatment of acute ischaemic stroke is becoming more widespread. There is a strict national guideline to adhere to (standardized inclusion/exclusion criteria, the use of National Institutes of Health stroke scale assessment prior to thrombolysis). Alteplase is the only tissue plasminogen activator licensed for this purpose in the United Kingdom. Although the absolute reduction in mortality in clinical trials has been very small, there is a significant morbidity benefit with a higher proportion of patients with good neurological recovery. Intense monitoring during and after thrombolysis is necessary, including blood pressure monitoring to look out for signs of cerebral haemorrhage and anaphylaxis – known complications associated with thrombolysis.

 KEY POINTS

- Stroke is a common medical emergency that carries high morbidity and mortality.
- The field of stroke management is rapidly evolving. It is important to be aware of the different types of stroke syndrome and their treatment algorithms.

History

A 52-year-old man has presented to his GP with a four-month history of back pain. This is associated with recurrent fever and weight loss of 4 kg over the previous four months. The back pain has been gradually getting worse and is now constant, radiating to the front of his chest. It is made worse on lifting and movement and is only mildly alleviated by paracetamol and ibuprofen. He is normally fit and well. He cannot recall any trauma or heavy lifting that might have triggered this pain. He was born in India and has not left the UK since becoming a resident in 1976.

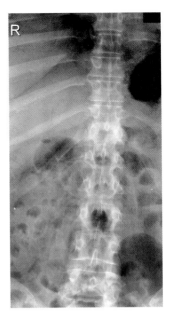

Examination

There is no lymphadenopathy. Cardiorespiratory, abdominal and neurological examinations are unremarkable. There is general tenderness around the thoracic spine extending down to the upper lumbar region. There is no neurological deficit. Rectal examination is normal. A chest X-ray reveals a calcified nodule in the upper zone. A spinal X-ray is shown in Fig. 98.1. Observations: temperature 37.5°C, heart rate 96/min, blood pressure 120/80 mmHg, SaO_2 99 per cent on room air.

Figure 98.1

INVESTIGATIONS		
		Normal range
White cells	14.0	$4–11 \times 10^9$/L
Haemoglobin	12.8	13–18 g/dL
Platelets	400	$150–400 \times 10^9$/L
Sodium	140	135–145 mmol/L
Potassium	3.9	3.5–5.0 mmol/L
Urea	4.0	3.0–7.0 mmol/L
Creatinine	76	60–110 μmol/L
Corrected calcium	2.3	2.2–2.6 mmol/L
C-reactive protein	38	<5 mg/L
Erythrocyte sedimentation rate	45	Male, age/2; female, [age+10]/2 mm/h

Question

• What are the possible causes of this man's symptoms and investigation findings?

This man has presented with back pain associated with 'red flag' symptoms. When evaluating back pain the red flags that are important to explore are:

- first back pain at age <20 or >55;
- non-mechanical back pain (stiffness at rest);
- thoracic back pain;
- past history of cancer;
- history or examination findings suggesting immunosuppression (e.g. oropharyngeal candidiasis, oral hairy leucoplakia, Kaposi sarcoma);
- systemic symptoms (e.g. weight loss, night sweats, fever, rigor);
- abnormal neurology (e.g. abnormal bowel and bladder functions, abnormal sensation and coordination, muscular weakness);
- structural spinal defect and severe localized tenderness, especially in the thoracic region.

For these scenarios, further investigations should be targeted to look for possible underlying infections or malignancy.

This patient's chest radiograph shows a calcified nodule in the upper lobe, indicating old primary tuberculosis. The spine radiograph in Fig. 98.1 shows partial collapse of T11 and T12 with loss of the intervening disc space. These findings and systemic symptoms raise the possibility of Pott's disease (spinal tuberculosis), although other infection or malignancies cannot be completely excluded. The possible findings of vertebral osteomyelitis on plain radiography are bony destruction, wedge fractures, lytic or sclerotic lesions. If spinal cord compression is suspected, an urgent MRI of the spine and urgent referral to spinal surgeons should be organized. Any delay could potentially increase the possibility of permanent disability. Infections in the spine tend to involve the intervertebral discs early, whereas malignancy tends to affect the vertebrae themselves, often sparing the discs.

Over 50 per cent of vertebral osteomyelitis is caused by *Staphylococcus aureus* and tuberculosis. Pott's disease is most common over the thoracic region and can extend over several segments and through intravertebral foramina into the pleura, peritoneum or psoas muscles. If tuberculosis is suspected then HIV testing should be considered, as TB is more common in immunocompromised people. MRI of the spine is particularly helpful to look for osteomyelitis, a paraspinal tumour or abscess and spinal cord compression. Histology or microbiology samples should be taken to confirm the diagnosis whenever possible. Treatment should be directed towards the underlying aetiology.

 KEY POINT

- It is important to enquire about the 'red flag' symptoms when evaluating back pain to ensure serious disorders are not missed.

History

A 48-year-old man has presented with recurrent vomiting after a large binge of alcohol intake 24 hours ago. Over the last hour he has become short of breath with a new dry cough. This is associated with severe epigastric pain which is constant and radiating towards his right chest. He is normally fit and well and has no past medical history.

Examination

This man looks unwell and is cool to the touch. His jugular venous pulse (JVP) is not seen. There is no lymphadenopathy. His pulse volume is reduced and his capillary refill-ing time is 4 seconds. There is crepitus felt on the skin around the neck extending to the chest wall. His chest is dull to percussion on the right. Auscultation of the chest reveals air entry bilaterally with reduced breath sound and a pleural rub on the right side. His upper abdomen is very tender with absent bowel sounds. An ECG reveals sinus tachycardia. Observations: temperature 37.8°C, heart rate 130/min, blood pressure 90/60 mmHg, respiratory rate 28/min, SaO_2 92 per cent on room air.

🔍 INVESTIGATIONS		
		Normal range
Arterial blood gas on room air:		
pH	7.28	7.35–7.45
PO_2	7.9	9.3–13.3 kPa
PCO_2	3.1	4.7–6.0 kPa
Lactate	8.0	<2 mmol/L
HCO_3	16	22–26 mmol/L
Base excess	−9	−3 to +3 mmol/L

Questions

- What are the differential diagnoses?
- How would you resuscitate this man?

ANSWER 99

This man is moribund and appropriate resuscitation should be instigated immediately. His breathing should be supported with oxygen and his circulation should be fluid resuscitated.

The differential diagnoses are cardiogenic, hypovolaemic or septic shock. Given this presentation, a normal ECG would be highly unlikely in cardiogenic shock. The history of recurrent vomiting, lower chest pain and subcutaneous emphysema – the Mackler triad – is highly suggestive of Boerhaave syndrome (spontaneous oesophageal perforation). Gastric contents spill over into the mediastinum to cause acute mediastinitis. Resuscitation should be goal-directed according to the Surviving Sepsis guidelines (http://www.survivingsepsis.org). It is important to keep the patient 'nil by mouth'. An urgent plain film or CT with water-soluble contrast often confirms the diagnosis. The timing of imaging is sometimes difficult in critically unwell patients and patients should be adequately resuscitated to minimize the chance of deterioration in transit and at the radiology department.

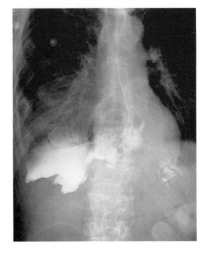

Figure 99.1

In this case a gastrograffin swallow confirms an oesophageal leak into the right chest cavity (see Fig. 99.1).

Other potential causes of oesophageal perforation are foreign-body ingestion and oesophageal instrumentation (e.g. oesophagogastroduodenoscopy, especially in preexisting oesophageal lesions such as cancers). Usually the patient is gravely ill. The abdomen may be rigid, leading to a false diagnosis of perforated duodenal ulcer. The pathophysiology of Boerhaave syndrome is not fully understood but the lack of serosa in the oesophagus increases the likelihood of rupture. Broad-spectrum antibiotics should be given immediately and urgent surgical review should be sought. The mortality of this condition is very high if it is not managed promptly and appropriately.

 KEY POINTS

- The definitive treatment for a perforated viscus is surgical intervention.
- It is important, however, to optimize the patient's condition prior to surgery through appropriate fluid resuscitation and antibiotic therapy.

CASE 100: NIGHT SWEATS, POLYURIA AND POLYDIPSIA

History

A 75-year-old man has presented to his GP with a four-month history of dry cough, reduced exercise tolerance due to exertional shortness of breath, and unintentional weight loss. These symptoms are associated with night sweats, polyuria and polydipsia. For the past week his urine has become very dark and discoloured. His history includes hypertension which was well controlled until four months ago. He does not smoke or drink alcohol. His drug history includes chlorthalidone, 50 mg once daily.

Examination

This elderly man is not icteric. There is no lymphadenopathy. Coarse inspiratory crackles are heard on auscultation of the lower zones bilaterally. There is clubbing of the fingers. Abdominal examination reveals a large right-sided varicocoele that does not collapse when lying supine. The rest of the examination is unremarkable. A chest X-ray is shown in Fig. 100.1. Observations: temperature 37.6°C, heart rate 104/min, blood pressure 190/110 mmHg, SaO$_2$ 94 per cent on room air.

INVESTIGATIONS		
		Normal range
White cells	12.2	4–11 × 10⁹/L
Haemoglobin	10.8	13–18 g/dL
Platelets	333	150–400 × 10⁹/L
Sodium	136	135–145 mmol/L
Potassium	3.4	3.5–5.0 mmol/L
Urea	10	3.0–7.0 mmol/L
Creatinine	120	60–110 (59–104 μmol/L)
C-reactive protein	415	<5 mg/L
INR	1.0	0.9–1.1
Corrected calcium	3.0	2.2–2.6 mmol/L
Urine	Blood 4+, protein 1+	

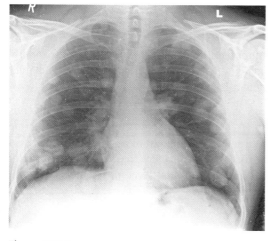

Figure 100.1

Questions

- What are the differential diagnoses?
- What further investigations should be performed?

The chest radiograph shows multiple, well-defined, rounded opacities that may explain his symptoms of shortness of breath and dry cough. Malignancies should be considered for multiple 'coin'-shaped opacities on a chest radiograph, especially when there are also complaints of night sweats and weight loss. Renal cell carcinomas are one of the most common sources of large pulmonary (cannonball) metastases. Sometimes it may be difficult to decide whether there is bacterial pneumonia that has superinfected the underlying malignancy, especially when there are pneumonic symptoms (fever, productive cough and shortness of breath) and raised inflammatory markers (which can be raised solely due to malignancy). If there is enough suspicion for superinfection then empirical antibiotics should be started.

The dark urine which may suggest macroscopic haematuria is a symptom of urological malignancy until proven otherwise, although rarely glomerulonephritis can present in this way. The classical triad for renal cell carcinoma or hypernephroma is macroscopic haematuria, loin pain and palpable mass. In reality patients rarely present with all three symptoms and signs. Hypernephroma may also present with microscopic haematuria, so this is a reason for investigation for possible underlying urological malignancy.

Varicocoeles are a common condition that affects 10 per cent of males. Ninety per cent of varicocoeles occur on the left and this may be due to the difference in venous drainage of the two sides. The left testicular vein drains into the high-pressure renal vein whereas the right testicular vein drains directly into the inferior vena cava. When these drainages are obstructed by tumours such as hypernephroma it may present as varicocoele. Such varicocoeles may not collapse when lying supine – a pointer towards further investigation for underlying invasive malignancy. A short history of varicocoele, especially on the right side, should also trigger further investigation for underlying malignancy.

The history of polyuria and polydipsia is consistent with the finding of hypercalcaemia. This should be treated with a combination of fluid resuscitation (normal saline) and furosemide in the first instance. Patients with this level of calcium are often dehydrated, so fluid resuscitation is essential. Although it may seem counterintuitive, the concurrent use of furosemide could also reduce hypercalcaemia through inhibition of calcium reabsorption in the ascending loop of Henle. If this regimen fails, then bisphosphonates should be considered. Hypercalcaemia is a poor prognostic sign as it may suggest bone metastasis or parathyroid-hormone-related-peptide secretion by hypernephroma cells. There are a number of other peptide hormones reported to have been secreted by hypernephroma cells: gonadotrophins, renin, insulin, erythropoietin and vasopressin. Other paraneoplastic conditions are fever, night sweats, cachexia, anaemia, amyloidosis, deranged liver function without liver metastasis, and polymyalgia.

The main investigation for hypernephroma is CT scan of chest, abdomen and pelvis for staging and to evaluate local anatomy. A bone scan should be considered if bone metastasis is likely, and mercaptoacetylglycine (MAG3) renogram may be used to assess differential renal function if chronic kidney disease is suspected. Needle biopsy is usually avoided as the diagnostic yield is low and it may risk tumour seeding. Radical nephrectomy is the treatment of choice for hypernephroma.

KEY POINT

- Hypercalcaemia is a common oncological emergency that should be screened for and treated appropriately.

INDEX

Note: References are in the form of case number with page numbers in brackets.